KISSED BY CANCER

YOU CAN SURVIVE AND THRIVE WITH HOPE HUMOR AND HUMILITY

SUE LACHMAN

JOIN MY VIP CLUB

Sign up for the VIP Club newsletter for your updates, book release details and your free books.

I will send you a free book: ***Rethinking Relationships***

Your FREE membership of my VIP Club newsletter will give you access to more free books and big discounts on my future releases. I'll keep you regularly update with all the latest news and you'll be the first to know when new books are coming out.

The VIP Club is a 100% spam-free zone

Go here:

https://www.suelachman.com/rethinking-relationships

To claim your Free Book '***Rethinking Relationships***'

INTRODUCTION

March 1986

It's such an emotional whirlwind.

On the morning after my wedding day, I looked in the bathroom mirror at the hotel where we were staying for our first night of marriage and muttered, "Now look what you've gone and done."

I loved my new husband, but this commitment was for life. I remembered my father's words minutes before he took me down the aisle: "Are you sure about this? It's not too late if you want to change your mind. I can take you home and sort it out."

I was shocked. Why on earth would I want to back out? I loved my fiancé so much. Now, however, my father's words rang in my ears. It dawned on me that just as the sun would rise, this man I loved would hopefully be by my side forever and a day.

There was no time to reflect or feel sorry for myself. We left for our honeymoon that morning. I was excited about flying to Florida to see Mickey Mouse. I admit I had encouraged Frank, and persuaded him that a holiday at Disney World would be a perfect start to our marriage.

At the end of the long nine and a half hour journey, we arrived safely. When they asked us at the airport why we were visiting America, Frank looked green. He kept his eyes on me and muttered under his breath, "I don't like flying."

Oops! Too late to tell me now, and you have the flight home yet to come!

It was fun. We laughed, ate, spent time enjoying each other's company and, of course, saw Mickey Mouse. Then for some reason, a few days into our honeymoon, I did a breast examination in the shower in that hotel in Orlando. I felt a lump.

How could I tell the man I had just married that I felt a lump!

I resolved to keep quiet until we arrived back in London. For the rest of the holiday I kept thinking that this might be my last holiday. I felt such turmoil inside but I knew that until I had proper testing it could be anything and not necessarily cancer. I decided this would not ruin our time together and put it aside. I can't say I didn't think about it, but whenever it came to mind I was not interested in entertaining it until we got home—to London.

One day after we landed in London, I told Frank about the self-examination. He took it in his stride and hugged me. He always looked like nothing was going to upset him – he was often quiet and calm whereas I was a live wire.

My mom was the next person to tell and I knew she had her own story. Now you've got to love my mom. She was one of twelve and one of her sisters had breast cancer at a young age. Not only that, but only five years earlier my mom had been diagnosed with cancer and was due to be operated on.

On the advice of a close friend, she visited a faith healer. I remember her telling me that he didn't touch her but put his hands just above her breast where the tumor was meant to be. She felt warmth flood her body and a deep feeling of calm washed over her. When she returned to the surgeon for all the pre-operation tests, they found nothing. It looked like the tumor had gone.

The operation never took place. She was healed.

When I told her about my lump she dived into action and started making doctors' appointments for me. Within a short time a doctor told me he needed to operate, so he could determine what was happening. He explained that if it was not cancer, he would sew me up and that would be the end of it. If, however, it was cancer, he would wake me and let me know my breast needed to be removed. That's how it was then: no choice. It was final, cut it off.

All this frightened my mom, reminded her of her sister's journey with cancer. At the doctor's appointment she asked me to leave so she could speak to him alone. I have no idea what they spoke about, although my guess is she told her story and that of my aunt.

My auntie Lily was one of the kindest, most loving people I have known. She was always there for me as a child. She bought my first doll, which was an extra special treat for me as my parents couldn't afford toys when I was young.

She was diagnosed with breast cancer and her breasts were removed long before I was born. I was made aware of her cancer when she was too ill to live alone and my parents brought her to our apartment to be with us.

We lived on the top floor of a large building apartment where there was no elevator. My father used to carry her downstairs if she needed to go anywhere. He told me that it wasn't difficult as she was so light. I had no idea that she had little time to live. It wasn't until she went into a hospice that I realized how serious it was. I was home from teacher training college and my mom and I were about to leave to visit my aunt. I took the phone call telling us that she had passed away. I couldn't believe it. I loved her so much. I was heartbroken. I still think of her and miss her.

Now here I was sitting with my mom and the doctor as a married thirty-one-year-old woman. Not a child! My respect for her and my trust and belief that she knew what was right to say struck me then and now. I knew she had my best interests at heart and I could see the funny side of being sent out of the room as though expelled from a classroom.

The operation took place. I have a pretty scar to show for it and a benign cyst was removed.

If the only thing people learned was not to be afraid of their experience, that alone would change the world.

Sydney Banks

How often are we scared of the future? Or should I say, what we think will be our future? Fear of the unknown concerns us, and we worry about things that might never happen.

I was fortunate to hear about the Three Principles for the first time in 2008. We had moved lock stock and barrel with our five children from London to Israel. I didn't hear what the principles were pointing to immediately, but incrementally they seeped into my psyche and I changed. I became more at ease and at peace with my life.

I now realized that seeing my husband and children as the root of all of my angst was something I had invented. I drew the same conclusions about the parents I helped when it came to fighting for the rights of their special needs children. I no longer saw them as the obvious cause of my frustration, worry and annoyance.

When I saw life differently, I understood that I am the creator of my own reality, not anyone or anything else. Still, could this knowledge, this understanding, really help me with the 'big stuff' in life? I would have to put it to the test. And what are these Three Principles?

The Three Principles explain how our experiences are created. All our experiences are generated from within. We can only experience anything via Thought, Mind, and Consciousness. They work in and around us whether or not we realize, understand or know about them. It is not an intellectual understanding we need to have. In fact, the more we attempt use our intellect to understand and work them out, the further away we get from grasping these Principles. Just like trying to get hold of cigarette smoke as it wafts towards us, it dissipates as we think we're reaching it and attempt to bring it towards us. Finally it eludes us.

I know that sounds crazy, but humor me for a minute, please. Principles are facts, truths. They don't change or waver; they're not passing. They're stable, solid, and grounded. They're constant, universal and neutral, whoever or wherever we are. Our whole life experiences work using these principles day in and day out without us knowing or doing anything.

Thought with a capital T is the power to be able to think, and we are thinkers. Our personal thoughts, the ones we have constantly in our mind, are what we are thinking in the moment and are fluid, always flowing through us. We often get seduced by our thoughts and believe them to be the truth. But truth is fact, certainty, and our thoughts are not made of truths and certainties.

Consciousness with a capital C is our ability to be

aware. Our senses inform us when we are conscious of something and bring our thoughts to life in 3D.

Mind with a capital M is the source of all energy that we're always connected to, even when it doesn't look that way. It's our minds that receive thoughts, closely followed by our opinions, beliefs, ideas and views: all of these are now personal to us as individuals.

I was guided by some of the top facilitators in this field and have come to see this for myself, so I don't take my thinking so seriously anymore. Having a sense of this doesn't mean that I will forever and a day be happy and will never take things to heart. I am not perfect; I still have feelings but I know they are not telling me I'm useless or can't do anything right.

They are merely informing me of what I'm thinking in that moment. Nothing else: not who I am, what I am, or where I am.

Knowing from a place deep within that I am resilient, that we all are resilient, and that I am always able to come back into alignment takes so much stress off me. It means that in everyday situations I don't need to look elsewhere, outside of me, in order to feel happy and content. There is no need for tools, strategies and techniques as we have everything we need all the time even when we don't see that clearly.

I am not the controller. As much as I might like to try and be in charge of what happens to me, life doesn't work that way. If I could I'm sure I would not have a cancer diagnosis. Acknowledging that there is an intelligence, a life force that is in control, means much of my thinking is taken off the table automatically. I can leave it all alone for the universe to deal with.

To illustrate this, here is a metaphor I heard at the Viva

event in 2015. Michael Neil, a well-known author and speaker, told this story to his students. One of them passed it on at the Viva event I attended and spoke at in 2016.

Viva is held in Albir, Spain, nestled along the coast between Alicante and Valencia. The event started in 2015 and was the brainchild of two wonderful women who dreamed of bringing about a feeling of community and love in a friendly, fun and light atmosphere whilst sharing an understanding of the principles that had so profoundly affected their lives and the lives of those who attended the annual event.

The story is about a young pilot who completed his training and was on his first solo flight. He was halfway through the flight when things started to go wrong. The plane lost altitude and kept veering to the right. He became anxious and scared. He gripped the controls, trying to turn things around and get out of what looked like an inevitable spin to the ground. He appealed to the control tower and reported that he was out of control and in a spin. The control tower replied: "Take your hands off the controls."

Spin recovery is not difficult. You need to break the stall on your wings and the plane will fly itself out of a spin. Reducing the throttle is of paramount importance although it is contrary to our thinking. Even though the pilot was panic stricken, the person in the control tower remained calm and gave instructions. The pilot didn't hear them at first – they were like a background hum that he didn't pay attention to. The hum grew louder. Thankfully, he finally received the message loud and clear. The minute he took his hands off the controls, the plane realigned. Then he was able to carry out the next necessary procedures to make sure he could fly back to his base.

That is a huge lesson for each and every one of us. We

are not in control. Our bodies, our minds have an inbuilt mechanism to right themselves without our interference. That is comforting, life changing, a relief.

June 8th

It's not death that frightens me but FOMO. Yes, I am scared to death of missing out on my son Yosef's marriage, my grandchildren growing up without me. Not being there, just an empty space where I was. I am scared and worried how my children with Down syndrome will cope without me. Will anyone come to the funeral, see my family mourning? Will I be able to follow their trails, will I be able to help them from on high or even from down there? What about the grandchildren I might never see? So many things.

Something happened on a Thursday when I poured my heart out to God. I told him that I was done trying new ways to get people to listen to anything I had to say about how my life was transformed and that a simple understanding of how life works could change anyone. I was done with trying this course or that course, feeling like I was getting closer, but not really. Constantly trying to learn new things so I could be heard in the jungle of online courses. No more doing. It was all too exhausting, even though I believed that my work was Godsent, that I had a duty to be sharing what I had seen.

I learnt how to produce an online parenting course and gave my complete love and time to it. All the small pieces that make up the whole took time and dedication. I thought I was meant to do that. Like a wheel going round, churning, the cogs moving slowly, I felt as though I was getting closer, then not! But closer to what? To making a fortune, to fame, to respect?

I prayed, no I begged for clarity, begged to know what to do, how to do it. What direction should I take? Should I continue but just with 1:1 clients or groups or retreats or... well what the heck do you want of me? Tell me, give me a sign. There it is, it popped into my head: 'Just gimme some kinda sign, baby'! However, it was not quite the same, as I think that very old song was asking some girl to give him a sign if she still loved him. My question was similar. It was more like: I have tried it all – I think I might be on the right track but now give me a helping hand. I need your guidance.

JUNE 9th

Friday morning I woke up and God's hands led me to do a breast examination. Yes, that sounds weird; I saw it happening, playing out in slow motion. I didn't feel as though I was doing anything, but I was being led to my right breast. I felt a lump; I checked the other breast to ascertain if it was normal and the same as the other side. I explored again, interested in its shape and length. I prodded to see if it hurt but it hurt as little or as much as the other breast which had nothing in it...or at least not a lump.

Calm reigned over me. That might sound surprising but

I had seen so much of this since my transformational adventure started over ten years ago. I know everyone experiences these moments, but we too often push them to the back of our minds as something that just happened or we attribute them to having an adrenalin rush or a similar belief. We forget those wonderful calm, warm, fuzzy feelings that wash over us, as if we are being carried and looked after. They're replaced by the old stale stuff that is in our heads and then they are gone.

Everything fell away. I had no thoughts about my life, just a bond, a feeling of unconditional love and peace. I knew I had to get the lump checked. I also knew I had to leave to go to see my eldest grandson in his end-of-year show. I love all that sort of thing. It's such fun to see a whole bunch of little men playing out their parts that they have worked on for so long. For me, this was our first, our eldest grandchild, something special. Excuse the pun, but my chest was full of pride knowing I was going to see him in his show.

First I had to speak to Frank. I needed to tell him my news and ask him to make an urgent appointment for a full breast examination. Deja vu: this was the second time I had to tell him I had found a lump in my breast. I left the house and so did the thoughts of me possibly having breast cancer. Frank stayed at home with his thoughts about the news I had given him.

I misjudged the timing of the journey and left very early. I had arranged to go to the apartment of Elliot and Goldie, my eldest son and daughter-in-law, and from there I would go to the show with Goldie and our latest grandchild, Talia, a beautiful little girl of two weeks. It was delightful. I got the gist, though my Hebrew is lacking. I loved the music and found myself tapping my feet and swaying to the rhythm. I bathed in the sheer love of life that the ten boys in front of me enjoyed. Yonatan, my grandson, sang at the top of his lungs and I felt I would burst with pride and happiness. Such a handsome young man, who I love more than words can ever describe. I'm unbiased, of course!

It was not until I was back home that I felt full of thoughts and worries. What if...? What will happen...? How will it all work out...? Will I be strong enough; will I survive? And I cried. I sobbed in private, tucking myself away in the bathroom until the tears stemmed. But I had no time; I had to get on. That day we were expecting eighteen guests for the Friday evening meal, with five of them staying in our house.

Our daughter, Chaya Gittel, was coming home from the apartment where she lives with four other girls, a house mother and other helpers. Elliot, Goldie and their three children were spending Shabbat with us. Alister, our second son, his heavily pregnant wife Yael and their daughter Yocheved were bussing it to our house and would be arriving soon. Yosef, our third son, was home from the Air Force along with a friend, someone we had known for years. Eighteen guests meant I needed to get on with things; life was happening. That was how it was for us. Our house was constantly full of visitors and I couldn't remember a time when Frank and I were alone on Shabbat.

On Friday evening, something terribly innocent happened. A highchair was moved and it touched my foot. It didn't really hurt; it only brushed my foot but I could feel the tears well up inside me and I rushed off to the bathroom to cry. Now was not the time to tell my family when there were so many others around. It was clearly on my mind somewhere and had come up to remind me.

Frank made a doctor's appointment for 2:30 p.m. on

Sunday afternoon. I was relieved, knowing I was due to see someone sooner rather than later. Little did we know what was to follow.

I realize now that the stress of thinking about what might happen brought on a cold with a vengeance. I could not breathe. My nose felt like it would never get enough air into it and I started coughing. My chest felt tight and each time I spluttered I ached. I am grateful that I know life goes on and my thoughts will ebb and flow because that is part of life. No matter that I am having stressful thoughts; they will go on their own, but the power of the thoughts made a physical impact on me.

Like a lot of other people, I stress out about things. The things I stress out about are often something from my past that is randomly brought up in my head. Why would I want to bring something up and make myself feel the stress as if it's all happening now? Sometimes I conjure up a path I think will happen in the future. I will work at it in my head until I have it just the way I think it will happen. I literally scare myself to death...or stress out with my fanciful thinking...and it hasn't even happened. What wonderful imaginations we all have. I can make up or bring back to life whatever I want, whether it really happened that way or not. I am the all-powerful 'Superthought Woman'. Wow! How cool is that? Except I scare myself silly.

Just like the ocean that comes in waves toward the beach, back and forth, with some crashing waves and some gentler, the busy chatter in our heads ebbs and flows. I thank God that I can see that internal chatter as just chatter sometimes. It doesn't mean that because I realize I have made up a load of stuff, including past memories, that I lack feelings. I sometimes experience them intensely. Some things have actually fallen away and I haven't seen them for a while. For the most part, I live in a place where I'm more able to sit back and observe rather than feel I always need to jump in and say and do things.

The only truth I can report in all of this is that I have breast cancer. At times I might think it's the end of the world and I might freak out about it, worrying that I might miss out on something. At other times I'm calm and know that I will survive. I'm good at composing what might happen but my moment to moment experience depends on my fluctuating thoughts.

June 11th

I woke Sunday morning intent on getting as much washing shoved into the machine as possible. After all, if you're dead you can't do the washing, and there were a lot of sheets and towels to get done. That is what went round in my head. I laughed because it was a ludicrous thought. I couldn't settle and it was interesting to me that when I realized my cleaner wouldn't be coming in I was able to switch so quickly into...get moving, clean! So that's what I did. I cleaned my downstairs until it shone. Now no one was allowed to walk anywhere and definitely not do any cooking.

My appointment was near and my stomach started to do cartwheels. It jumped up and down, getting into position then very carefully performing the perfect cartwheel. First the hands in the position on the floor, then the legs one after the other in exact alignment with toes pointed. Internally it didn't feel good. I felt uncomfortable. My insides were complaining and frankly I need the bathroom more than usual when my body reacts to extreme nerves.

Frank drove me to the local appointment. A short journey. The receptionist at the doctor's surgery looked at her computer and told me that I didn't have an appointment for a breast expert. She had no idea what I was talking about. There was some mix up, as Frank knew he had made an appointment and explained on the phone who I needed to see. But there was no one there to examine me, and she explained that that doctor doesn't come in on Sundays.

Frank appeared confused. The receptionist looked strangely at me but pointed me to the room where the doctor would see me. We waited for a moment as a woman went into the room. She nodded toward me, giving me permission to enter. Sitting at the desk was a man who barely looked up. He explained that the woman was a student nurse. I remarked, "I'm glad there's a woman in the room." His eyes went to the ceiling. Well, I'm sorry, but I wanted a woman in the room!

The student nurse nodded and looked at me as if she had been trying to put compassion in her eyes. She said nothing. I felt I needed to qualify my statement.

"Not that I mind a man, but it's nice to have a woman present."

The doctor stared at his computer.

"What can I help you with, Susan?"

My parents used to call me Susan, as do my sister Amanda, brother Anthony and other relatives, but I have been Sue more years than Susan, so for some reason I felt like giggling. I explained about the lump. He told me he was a gynecologist so he couldn't help me – I needed to see a breast surgeon urgently. However, he would take notes and then give me the necessary paperwork. He gave me a couple of options on the route to take. I could make a further appointment at the clinic with a specialist doctor who would be able to examine me, or I could call a hospital directly to try and make an appointment for a specialist to see me.

"Which side?"

"Right."

He went on to ask a myriad of questions. Does it hurt? How big is it? When did you find it? Is your skin smooth or not? Is there discharge from the nipple? Does it hurt when you touch it? All these I answered as best as I could and yet he still looked at his computer. The next question flummoxed me.

"Where did you have your last mammogram?"

I couldn't remember the name of the place, however much I racked my brain. Then I said the name of something which I promptly remembered had a similar meaning to the word for giving birth...I thought the name of the place was something along those lines. He stopped, still looking at his computer. I looked at the student nurse, who still had those eyes.

Does she practice this, 'I understand, dear' look? She said nothing. Then my head cleared and I wanted to laugh. It was hilarious. Here I was sitting with someone who only looked at his computer and someone else who said nothing but had 'understanding practiced eyes'.

I bet you would look if I had come in with a complaint you could look at. Not to be too crude, but if you needed to look inside me, well that would be different; then maybe you would acknowledge me sitting here.

The next thought was too funny and I had to stop myself from laughing out loud. I did mention that it was funny that I had said completely the wrong name of the place where I had my last mammogram, but he was looking at his computer and her head was on one side with those eyes and closed mouth.

The moment passed. I held myself from laughing, got the papers and went outside to see my husband. We went to the desk to get an appointment to see a breast surgeon at the clinic. The receptionist was not able to contact her so they took my number and said they would call me, hopefully that day or the next.

We went home no closer to knowing what was what but that one of the options the doctor had given us could still be explored. I called a hospital with the name of a surgeon the doctor had suggested and asked for an urgent appointment.

"24th of July," she told me.

"Hold on a moment. What date in July? Did you know this is urgent? That means I would have to wait over a month for an appointment and it might be too late by then. Could you repeat to me, is this the only appointment you have for something that is urgent, even privately?"

Yes that was it...a dead end.

Isn't it strange how we can feel so helpless, so vulnerable, so not in control. I felt in limbo, not knowing what to do, and then suddenly something came to mind. I would call a family friend, Avital, the eldest of five children who moved in two doors away from us when we were living back in London. She worked as a radiologist in the hospital that I couldn't remember the name of...she might have a solution and a doctor who might see me quickly.

I felt calm in that moment, knowing deep down that this would be sorted sooner rather than later. I WhatsApped Avital and asked her to keep it quiet until I had some time to speak to our boys, Elliot, Alister and Yosef.

"I need to speak to you but it's confidential," was the message I sent her. I don't know why, but I was off guard when she called me and I picked up to speak to her. I suddenly felt very teary and choked up. I could hardly speak.

"Breathe slowly, tell me what it is," she said.

I told her the story and as I did, I immediately got back in alignment and was able to continue, even joking about something during the conversation. Something positive happened: a feeling of being enveloped in love and care and that it would be sorted, it would be okay no matter what.

Within a few days she had organized an appointment for a mammogram and then set up an appointment for a breast and lymph node biopsy. I hadn't even considered the idea of needing a biopsy on the lymph nodes, although I had some tell-tale signs that they might be involved without realizing until sometime later. I read somewhere and heard first hand from a friend who had breast cancer that there is an odor similar to what we term B.O. (body odor) emanating from our armpits. Even when we have cleaned under our arms and put on deodorant the smell is strong. I noticed this in my body, although initially I did not put two and two together.

The ins and outs of what, when and how are not all relevant. I just knew that the following day I was due to have a mammogram and wondered if I should tell my children. I was weighing this up when I realized they needed this information; this was not a secret and I just knew they would be okay inside even if sometimes it might not look that way to them or me. I should add that the decision I made to tell my family and friends, in fact the world, is my decision that I feel is right for me. That does not mean that others have to do the same: it's not right or wrong.

I initially made sure they were at home in a 'safe' environment, whatever that means. I called Alister, my second son, to ask him where he was. He was at home so I tried to tell him, but the tears came and I couldn't speak. I handed the phone to Frank, who was also lost for words and really didn't know what to say until I pulled myself together.

Then, with a much stronger voice and a feeling of being able to accomplish this and anything else that came my way, I told him about my experience since Friday.

Having told one son I thought it was fair and wise to tell them all. I gingerly called Elliot, my eldest son, having in the back of my mind the fact that he usually worked from home on a Monday. I told him and then my third son, Yosef. There is no point in saying anything to our two youngest in the family because they might not understand.

My sister and brother were next. My sister, always the one hoping for the best, told me it might be just a cyst. She was right, of course, but it doesn't stop the fear that it might be serious. My head was also filling with random erroneous thoughts accusing me of being the cause of whatever will happen as a result of something I had done in the past.

What can I say about the mammogram? It's painful and even more so when there is a tumor. I survived it.

I'm once again in a state of flux, waiting for the next part to unravel. It has been confirmed from the mammogram that there is something there to take seriously and I will need an ultrasound and a biopsy. I hoped that I would not need to have a biopsy, although I knew from past experience that I would need a follow up of an ultrasound after a mammogram.

So as I wait, going in and out of fear and worry, I think of what I want to do as soon as possible to spend my time with my family, to enjoy them and to enjoy life as it is for this moment. I cry sometimes at the thought of not knowing and I feel relief at other times that I have such a wonderful family. I do want to say this, however controversial some might think it is.

I concerned myself for most of my life with what people would think of me. How I looked to people, whether I'd said the right thing. Would it be in alignment with what others think? At one stage I believed that shouting and being out there, being brutally blunt even to the extent of being rude was the way to go, but underneath I was always terrified of rejection. If anyone ever tells you that you can be happy all the time, it's not true. If anyone says that you will never be stressed or overwhelmed, it's not correct...run a mile from them.

Yes, you can change. All of us can be different; we shift every minute of the day, in and out of one mood or another, from one thought to another just like that, in the blink of an eye. If we suppose and expect there is somewhere to get to, something to do, we are taken away from the simplicity of life and fall into the misunderstanding that society has made us believe is the right way. We end up full of thoughts running amok in our heads and taking them as gospel truth. They are not the truth, they are not constant. God is constant, the Universe is constant. We come and go, our thoughts come and go and we go in and out of calm, in and out of being sad and happy and all the bits in between.

If there is something I would love people to hear, it is this: every moment you are worried or anxious about anything, it takes you away from being grateful for what you have. I know that might sound flippant because I am very aware that those anxious feelings are compelling and real, but just know that all our feelings are always just coming from our thoughts in that moment. Nothing else.

The unknown was most definitely the scary part of life for me at one stage. We always consider we need to know everything and then try and control the situation or people. It still catches me unaware even though I have become much more at ease and go with the flow.

Now it was time for a biopsy.

The most interesting thing for me was that my body was taking the news about the tumor differently to how my mind was. My body and my mind were not reacting in a similar manner. I felt calm and put together but my stomach thought differently. Somewhere along the line a nervous thought was literally manifesting itself through my stomach. At the end of the procedure I had to make a huge dash to the toilet. I felt like a baby, as if I was going to soil myself during the last moments whilst they sorted the wounds out.

I cannot describe the gratitude I have towards Avital, who sat there calmly next to me throughout the whole ordeal. I grabbed her hand, squeezing tightly in particular when they began cutting and the anesthetic hadn't started to work. Her easy going, sensible kindness put me at ease. We all knew it was cancer but we had to wait for confirmation. As I finally came to sit next to Frank, he gently took my hand.

The results were due in a couple of weeks. Avital was already busy at work and was told that when we got the initial results we could see the breast surgeon. Usually people have to wait for two parts of the story to come back but I officially had someone who was able to help me from the inside. It's not always what you know, but who you know.

A few days later, we met for lunch. Our family together. My three oldest boys, their wives and the two babies. The other children were in school and this gave us time to talk with little interruption. I was greeted with hugs from everyone. There was a sadness about the outcome and inevitable treatment I would soon embark on. There was also a wonderful feeling of love and support. The tears came and went; we joked and laughed. We arrived separately but left as one.

Then I took to Facebook. I didn't want to hide anywhere. People, including me, have no idea what it means to have cancer until we experience it ourselves. (It is written without checking the spelling or the grammar but as it came out from the heart and with honesty in all its rawness.)

It was important for me to tell my close friend Joyce about the diagnosis and I invited her for lunch. I felt choked when it was time to tell her; it was difficult to get the words out. It was all still very raw for me, and hearing the words, "I have breast cancer" scared me. But quietly, gently, before I was able to say the words, she said, "Whatever it is Sue, we will work it out." That was my cue to tell her between my tears. We spent time with a wonderful feeling of being connected and full of love. I am grateful for that time and the shared togetherness I experienced in those moments.

June 22nd – FB post

For those who understand, please say Tehillim* for me. I never thought I would be doing this, but here I am asking for your prayers, your help to storm the heavens and ask Hashem (God) to help me. I can only ask and so can you. I had a mammogram and a biopsy and am waiting for the results for a lump in my breast and in my lymph nodes under my arm.

This was my first post on Facebook, letting people know about my inevitable cancer diagnosis.

*Tehillim are Psalms.

June 26th – FB post

My results are back but unopened. Have an appointment to see a breast surgeon tomorrow morning. SOOOOOO until the envelope is opened the result can still be changed for the better.

I AM VERY CALM at the moment, thinking about it very little in fact. Not using any deodorant as one of my lymph nodes has a lump so I tried coconut oil. Now all my thinking is about how I smell like I'm cooking something...

I see more and more that even when I feel low, there is still beauty to be found. I look outside and see the stunning blue sky and breathe the air. I am alive even though sometimes it feels like I am drowning.

Frank and I met Avital at the hospital when we went to see Dr. Olsher, the breast surgeon. Avital came armed with the envelope housing the first and important part of the results. Although I had given her permission to open the envelope before we met, she declined and I can't say I blame her. Dr. Olsha examined me and gently but professionally explained what would happen in order. He had a wonderful bedside manner, mixed with just the right amount of professionalism. I felt safe and cared for.

June 27th – FB post

I would like to thank you all for your prayers, kind words, good deeds and love you have sent me. Today my results came back and I have breast cancer and cancer in my lymph nodes. I will need chemo, an operation and radiotherapy. We are still waiting to find out what stage cancer I have and other details. They need the second part of the results to see exactly what treatment will be needed but there is now an outline of a plan.

.   .   .

I WILL NEED to see an oncologist and was referred to Professor Cherny, who will schedule the chemotherapy and advise me of the type of drugs they will use and the number of treatment sessions for each drug. Before anything else they want me to have another mammogram at the hospital, so they have all the paperwork together in one place. They also want me to have a PET CT scan, which will scan my body to see if the cancer is anywhere else.

So now on to seeing to all the paperwork. It's a learning curve to make sure we have all the right documents. My fear is to turn up at an appointment and have the wrong papers with me. But I know all I can do, we can do, is our best.

The system here in Israel is confusing. A referral is given and then you need to take it into your preferred clinic and they approve the procedure and location for testing. They can refuse or send you to a more cost effective place. For a cancer diagnosis, the clinic we joined when we first came to Israel in 2006 agrees that all treatment and tests can be under the auspices of one hospital rather than using various hospitals in different locations. The exception is for the radiotherapy, where at the time of writing this, the facility does not exist in my approved hospital. Once your request is approved you receive a document confirming that the health clinic will reimburse the hospital.

I cannot count the journeys backward and forward that poor Frank made between our home and the local doctor's clinic. Often, he needed to advise the clinic as to the necessary paperwork. You either self-advocate or end up with the wrong paperwork only to be sent home by the hospital.

July 4th – FB post

Sitting waiting for my PET CT scan.

MORE IMPORTANTLY, we arrived with, yes you guessed it...the wrong paperwork. The paperwork was checked and rechecked with Avital. She even had it checked by someone in the department before we arrived. We were requested to fax it (can you believe that to this day they still use fax machines here to send and receive paperwork?) to the PET CT scan department and yet again, no one spotted anything wrong.

It all caught up with me. I cried and the receptionists immediately went into action and told me it would all be okay. Avital was out at a training day, so I couldn't even get her help and we had to wait. We made frantic calls to our local clinic doctor, where the nurse was really trying to help, along with the hospital receptionist. But my whole world was rocking. I felt on uneven ground, as if I couldn't find my balance, and I wanted to run and hide. The only thing that kept me calm was knowing that at the end of the day it would be how it was meant to be and I was not in control of this or anything else.

Then, it all suddenly came together and the fax that hadn't come through was emailed and the paperwork was there. Now all I had to do was sit and wait for my name to be called. Finally, it was my turn. I was taken first to one station, where they put a cannula in my arm. Then I was taken to a room where everything was explained. They were very kind and luckily spoke English well...phew!

I would have some nuclear medicine pumped into my body initially and then I would be taken to a nuclear shelter where every ten minutes I would be required to drink a fluid they put on the table next to me. Before the scan, I would need to empty my bladder.

So the nuclear medicine was started and in front of me was a small machine which made a clicking noise that progressively got louder. It was a Geiger counter.

"Just like the movies," I said to the guy who was concentrating on making sure it was all going to plan. He laughed. I thought it was really funny hearing the clicking and popping of the machine. Once I was radioactive, I entered the shelter. There were three open plan cubicles with a reclining chair in each and a table next to each chair. Now I could just relax and drink the liquid placed next to me.

The actual scan was easy. No undressing, fully clothed (thankfully) and fairly quick after the whole process before. One thing ticked off the list. Now the wait to see if it's anywhere else lurking in my body in hidden crevices that I might never be aware of.

At moments on some days my mind went all over the place... What if...then what, how would I? Many thoughts came in and went out. Some days some of them stayed for a while even though they were unwelcome. Other days and times I was calm, knowing that whatever would be, would be. I had little chance to change anything and I was in the hands of God and needed to go with the flow. Still, the stories we create can seem so real and terrifying; certainly mine are at times.

We never know how we might react whatever the news, diagnosis, trauma, but still we conjure up our own movies and live through them as if they are a given, the truth. It hasn't even happened and yet we act as if it has. So, bring out the popcorn, sit back and watch the movie, because that's all it is: we are writing a script of how we think it will be.

We had made arrangements to go to England as we had a wedding to attend in the north, in Manchester, on Sunday. We planned on flying out to London on the Thursday, spending the Sabbath with my sister Amanda, her husband Moy, my niece Orly, her husband and three children and my nephew Sammy and his wife. I hoped also to see my brother Anthony and his wife and son. Now we had another reason to be there. I wanted to see my sister and brother and spend time with them. We had made all the arrangements and just hoped we would be able to spend the time before seeing the oncologist.

July 6th – FB post

At airport. Off to see my family before I return to hear full results and treatment plan. What a motley crew. Can't help giggling. I try not to stare at a young man with runny glue coming off his front hair piece.

. . .

ISN'T that the spice of life? Isn't being able to look around and find the lightness in life the fun? We spend all too much time worried about how we need to be perfect and find out why we are not enough. Yet laughing, seeing the small simple things in life is where it's at. In those moments when we throw our heads back in abandonment, throw caution to the wind, we are fully in life. Nothing else matters.

That weekend was very special. We shared many tears for the journey ahead and many laughs. I felt the special bond with my family; their love and warmth surrounded me. There were unspoken words. A time to be together before embarking on the unknown road.

July 11th – FB post

I have just spent a very special weekend with my family. Lots of laughter, some tears (mainly me!) and loads of love and fun.

Now back into things and more news. Something was spotted on the PET CT scan I had last week. Something on my shoulder

(looks like my ego follows me everywhere). Tomorrow I have to have an MRI. Then off for full results and how to move forward with treatment on Thursday. Now first question is...am I claustrophobic?...hmmm, not sure – guess I will have to wait and see. Second question is...actually a statement – time for the medical marijuana.

I HADN'T EVER BEEN in a situation where I was concerned about being in a small tight place. Guess I will soon know when I go for the MRI. This was all new to me.

July 12th – FB post

Just on way home from MRI after midnight. Could not believe the noise of the machine even with headphones on. At least it's done and I was probably in there for at least forty minutes. Though could have made that up lol.

Tomorrow oncologist and another mammogram and the journey goes on.

AVITAL MET us for this first MRI and walked me through the process, which included a lengthy form. A cannula, yet another one, was set up ready for the dye to go in once I was on the table. I had to lie in a certain position and was told I must not move. I was strapped onto the bed and told to breathe normally. No deep breaths allowed. Now what do you do when you are told to do that? Well, am I the only rebel? Come on, I know you would do the same – want to breathe deeply or feel the need to. It was difficult in particular as the strap was across my chest and felt restrictive. In the end I started counting as I couldn't hear the music they put on.

Apart from the noise of the machine, and with headphones on, I felt my knee twitching. I was unceremoniously spoken to through the speakers.

"Are you okay?" they called.

"Yes," I replied.

"Then why are you moving?"

I didn't feel the need to answer. I was not sure how to stop anything in my body from twitching after being placed in a fixed position for any length of time.

July 13th – FB post

Another day at the hospital. Have been there since 12:30 p.m., now nearly 5 p.m.

Had another mammogram – ouch – and an ultrasound – ouch – that also hurt.

Went to see oncologist but he couldn't get results yet from MRI so back we go on Sunday. Also, my biopsy needs to go to a different lab and that will take about ten days.

Feeling okay with all of this and know there is still time to pray for good results from MRI.

IT WAS STARTING to feel as though the hospital was my second home.

July 16th – FB post

Woooooo hooooooooooooo!

I don't have the cancer in my bones! I have stage 2 breast cancer, which is also in my lymph nodes.

I start chemo which will be every three weeks on Sunday 23rd July. I will have eight loads of chemo, then an operation and radiotherapy at end.

Thank you to everyone for your prayers, thoughts, support and challah baking. Please keep me in mind as I start the treatment.

It's been an interesting journey. Some crying, some laughing and many internal conversations. I have laughed sometimes at the ridiculousness of some of the stuff in my head, full of doom and gloom, yet I knew deep down that I didn't have bone cancer.

Might have a hissy fit every so often but I'm singing.

. . .

OUR FIRST ENCOUNTER with the oncologist was pleasant. He told us that he too once had cancer. He slowly explained the results of the scans, which did indeed show there was something in my shoulder bone, but it might have been from an old injury. As I had broken both my wrist and elbow on that arm, it was possible the injury showed up as a potential cancer marker. He assured us there was nothing to be concerned about and he regarded it as not cancerous.

July 18th – FB post

Having breast cancer stinks!!!!!

First I had a biopsy which I seriously was not a fan of. They took bits from my breast and from my lymph node.

Then I had a PET CT scan where I hummed and was put in a nuclear shelter and then put into a doughnut for at least half an hour with my hands above my head – no moving allowed.

Then I had an MRI for my shoulder when they thought I had cancer in my shoulder bone – where I felt like my head was being drilled and I wasn't allowed to move for about 45 minutes.

Now I am having treatment on Sunday and they want me to return to put something in my breast instead of taking it out. I have to go back the next day after my first chemo. Really?!!! And they want me to have another MRI, this time on my breast.

GIVE ME A BREAK ALREADY!!!!!

I also have to dance around the fact that I want to get a license for medicinal marijuana and only certain people will give me a prescription even though it's my right.

HISSY FIT – 1? (who is counting?)

July 23rd – FB post

First chemo is postponed until tomorrow.

Chemo in the morning.

Procedure in the afternoon to put in a titanium wire to monitor the tumor for surgery if and when needed after chemo.

An all-day affair! Thanks to the nurses in the oncology department and the breast health department for putting the two together.

EXPERIMENT: shaved one side of head and left other to see the difference. #3 son says both sides will hurt as it's to do with the hair follicles whether shaved or not...let's see. Might help others make a decision in the future.

July 24th – FB post

Feeling vulnerable. In the hands of God.

SOMETIMES I JUST KNOW THERE is nothing to do, nowhere to go. Feeling vulnerable used to freak me out. It meant that I would show everyone that really I was scared and that I couldn't cope. No way would I put my heart on my sleeve for all to see. Then I saw something different and I realize that actually vulnerability is a place of strength and not weakness. It does not mean I am useless, unworthy. It just means in that moment I am feeling uncertain and not the dictionary definition.

'*Someone who is **vulnerable** is weak and without*

protection, with the result that they are easily hurt physically or emotionally.'

Collins Dictionary

If that were true then why did I feel protected and actually strong, not weak? Certainly, the thought of being vulnerable might bring me to believe that I am emotionally and physically shot. But then for that to be a truth it would happen to everyone ALL the time, and it doesn't.

It is to some extent a strongly held belief that feeling vulnerable is a bad thing. Society tells us that it is not good to be vulnerable: you are open to attack and could be badly wounded.

But what if it just says what's on the tin? Today, at this moment, I am feeling vulnerable. Nothing more, nothing less, except what we make up to fit into our belief system. Hold fire. Step back. It's just a moment in time. Maybe you will see it differently in a little while, maybe not.

Humor me and listen to this suggestion. It might not always be bad to feel vulnerable. We do not run the world – a jolly good thing that we're not in charge! We don't need to know everything all the time, and the realization that we don't know what might happen and how we will respond brings us to feel vulnerable.

Before the treatment started, the nurse from the oncology department made an appointment to see us to explain the system and what would happen each visit. Frank and my son Yosef came with me. One of the things she told me was to stop work.

"Whatever you are doing, stop," she said. "Don't get excited about cleaning and cooking."

Hold on, stop this record. Who gets excited about cleaning and cooking? Keep listening. She told me my treatment would impinge on everything in my life. Things won't be the same. Huh, really? Well that won't happen…

Until it did.

As part of the treatment, I had to get a couple of drugs. One was to be taken an hour before the infusion and the other to be taken afterward.

First stop with a prescription was to go to the nurse who works for our doctor. She told us we would need to go to the main office and make contact with the manager of that branch. We walked over to see the manager in charge of the health clinic. She told us she had no time to speak to us but I insisted. I told her I had been advised to see her and make sure she knew I had cancer and would need medications every so often. She was very short with me, as if she lacked the time of day. I was surprised but followed her instructions to go to the pharmacy and put the prescription in.

Next stop, the pharmacy. There we were informed that I was not eligible to get any discount on the drugs as I was not in the system. We relayed the instructions to the pharmacist. He immediately told us to follow him as he would speak with the manager, so back we all went to speak to the manager to sort it out.

Back at the main branch, the pharmacist spoke to the manager, insisting that she help us. Finally, she telephoned her boss, who put me into the system. Once that was done it was plain sailing. Why wasn't it done the first time?

What I do know is that the manager we spoke to was up to her ears in work. Her desk was covered in files and papers and she was constantly on the phone. Her head was full with other things and had not switched over to what I needed until someone came who knew the system and confronted her. We all get like that from time to time.

July 24th – FB post

First part of treatment in…was bright red. Had to suck ice whole time. Horrid taste in mouth. Now on to a clear liquid but feel freezing cold from sucking all the ice.

FOR THIS FIRST TREATMENT, although they took blood, I didn't have any results from the time before to wait for. So we started earlier than most in the room, who had to wait for about ninety minutes for their blood results to return and determine whether they could continue treatment.

So, this time it was a blood test, putting in the cannula for the day, being weighed and taking my height. Once I was settled into one of the comfy chairs around the room, it was a waiting game for the doctor to sign off on the medicine, but I understand that patience is the order of the day. Not only this day, but every day I am reminded about being patient. Waiting without any expectations.

It was a really weird sensation, with the liquids going through a tiny tube leading into my arm and then going to kill the cells. Yup, every cell. The good, the bad and the ugly. It was cold and immediately gave me this revolting metallic taste in my mouth.

It was evident with all the things going on that the process we had started for our son to go into assisted living accommodation should now become something of great importance. Not only does he not like me being ill in any way and fusses over anything out of order, but my hospital visits were already challenging. Our daughter had been in assisted living for some time and Refoel had seen her happy and content. He often told us that he wanted to go like her and be in an apartment with other boys. I needed to speak to his social worker.

"Hi. This is Sue Lachman, Refoel's Mum. How are you?"

"I'm fine. Thanks."

"I have something that I need to tell you which you will see makes Refoel's move into an apartment a little more urgent than before. I have breast cancer."

"Oh. I'm sorry to hear that. I will arrange it all."

She put the phone down before I could say anymore. Within five minutes she called me back.

"I'm so sorry," she said. "I was in shock to hear your news and didn't know what to say."

We discussed the options. This particular social worker was amazing. She was always willing to help and even if she was not available, she would call or email back within twenty-four hours. The previous social worker was hardly at work. It was difficult to get in touch with her and because she had so much time off from work, her case load was huge. Leaving messages or trying to call led us down dead ends. It meant that the official tests that were required to assess both Chaya Gittel and Refoel were never done.

The first port of call was to have Refoel retested. The first and only test was completed on our arrival in Israel and no longer reflected his needs. He was five when we moved to Israel from London and was now sixteen. The social worker set the ball rolling. We made an appointment to complete the necessary paperwork, followed by a meeting with a psychiatrist, a doctor and a different social worker from the center where he was assessed to determine his needs.

We were fully supported by our local social worker, who attended the meetings with us. The conclusion of the examinations showed that he would be eligible to live in an apartment. After all, why would he want to be home with two old people who were really not much fun? Rather he should be with others to be encouraged to be more independent and live his life to its fullest.

The main problem for moving our son was not when but where. Refoel is still in school and will be until he is twenty-one. We chose Seeach Sod not only for its impeccable reputation but also because they had the facility to help children from infancy into adulthood and old age. Part of their program involves acquiring apartments for six young people with special needs to live in alongside a bank of helpers who are with them when they are not in school or working.

But there were no vacancies. They applied for a license to include more young adults and we waited along with them for government approval. We were faced with a dilemma. Some of my appointments were late at night. On one occasion we had to ask Elliot to sleep over, leaving his wife and three children so he could be with Refoel and put him to bed. The other possibility was for him to be sent to the respite facility also available through Seeach Sod. We felt this was not a solution but putting a band aid on, and would be more disruptive for him, even though he loved it there.

The other alternative was for him to go into something run by the local authority. This was a much larger, more institutional set-up which we did not want for Refoel. Although we know he would have been well cared for, we all knew that something smaller and more personal would best suit him.

We did not know a new apartment close to our home would be an option that presented itself. It already had three young men; they were older than our son, but their mental age was the factor to consider, not their chronological age – that was irrelevant. We met with all the people involved in the housing department, who realized the urgency and also knew that this apartment would be an excellent fit for him.

It was set up very quickly for us to visit the apartment with our son and then wait for the completion of the paperwork. None of this could have been sorted out without my daughter-in-law Goldie. She was the guiding light, the person who was with us every step of the way, negotiating as well as speaking to all the moving parts and translating for us.

We wanted him to have stability, security and permanency. He needed to feel loved and yet still be able to come home. This was the perfect answer. He was excited about the prospect of living in the apartment and packed some of his belongings. It was a relief.

July 24th – FB post

Feeling woozy.

Had procedure where they put a titanium wire in my breast. First in went anesthetic, then he put a machine – it was sort of shaken (not stirred lol) and that was it...took all of a few minutes.

Now I'm wired.

IT IS AMAZING how clever it is that they can shoot a wire into my breast. I am in awe of man's capabilities. A tiny wire was literally shot into me. I didn't feel any pain, although the doctor warned me that I would feel a rocking sensation.

July 26th – FB post

Yesterday, Tuesday, was not such a wonderful day. I felt very weak, could even hear it in my voice when I spoke to someone. Worst of all I felt nauseous all the time so couldn't eat and needed to eat to take the steroids (which I really didn't want to take).

I did take the steroids later but was told that eating was necessary and take them earlier in the day as they might keep me awake. I slept well.

But here's what not everyone knows. There's a possibility of getting mouth sores. I have to use a soft toothbrush so as not to bleed in my mouth. Clean my teeth each time after eating.

I have to wash my mouth out several times during the day with warm salt water. I have to make sure my temperature does not go above 38 or go to hospital if it does.

I found it incredibly difficult to swallow anything hard without continuously sipping water.

This morning I feel weak still. I find it hard to stand for any length of time. Even walking is slow and carefully (especially with my history of broken bones!).

I want to give a shout out to Susan the nurse in the Breast Health department at Shaare Zedek hospital who kindly and thoughtfully WhatsApped me last night and then took the time to call me!! Thank you for your kindness and time to be there for me.

I AM WELL SUPPORTED by my family, close friends and the staff I am in closest contact with from the hospital. I know that if I need to ask anything, they will respond fairly quickly.

It was around this time that I became more aware of a couple of virtual Facebook friends who also had a diagnosis of breast cancer. Although all at different stages and levels of treatment, we started to be in touch. We encouraged each other through the tough times and laughed together. We were there for each other. Maureen and Kay, thank you for your friendship. It means so much to me to have gone through this experience with two wonderful human beings and be a part of the 'three amigas', as we call ourselves.

Apart from virtually, one of my visitors, Rachel, a previous client, came every Friday with a different bowl or platter of delectable food. She also spent time sitting and conversing.

For me, having visitors when I was weak from the chemo and unable to get out and about was a lifesaver. The human need to communicate, to feel loved, surfaced for me. When I was able, I wanted company, even if only for a short while.

Joyce, a good friend of mine, and her sister-in-law Naomi came weekly. Sometimes we went out for a short walk and sat in the town center, so I could see life from a different place than my rocking chair. At other times we sat in my lounge and chatted about nothing in particular. I was bowled over that they came one morning before 7 a.m. and accompanied me throughout the day when I went to hospital for treatment. Sitting with them, often in silence, was helpful. I have no words to express my thanks to them, but for them to know I love them for being there.

Others tended to stay away for a while.

I belong to a club called 'Experience' for over fifty-fives. I always joke with them that I am the youngest member, as most are in their seventies. At first I didn't receive many visits from members, but eventually at least once a week someone came. Those times helped the days go faster, filled with love and kindness.

One other visitor who helped so much was Devorah. She lives close by, although at the time I first met her, when I was still back in London, she was living in the north of England, in Manchester. We met when I traveled up there for work. She is an easy person to be with. Always chatty and funny. We have shared some serious moments too.

I want to thank her from the bottom of my heart for making me feel like a human being during my treatment, and giving me a manicure. She did this willingly, arriving with all her gear, and would take no money from me. On one occasion when she came to give me another manicure, I cried. I had had enough of my body, feeling like it was constantly pummeled. Sometimes it's easier to cry with a friend than your close family. They're able to step outside and just be with you.

Once again, Joyce and her sister-in-law Naomi came to visit and took me out for a walk. Shaky, I was hardly able to move; I needed someone by my side all the time. Joyce went into the ice cream shop for iced coffee. In my excitement to be out in the air and see people I drank it with relish, forgetting that dairy was not my friend. I was not well that night and some of the next day. Stomach pains were almost unbearable at times.

July 30th – FB post

In the face of all sorts of things coming at you, how do you hold on? What is it that keeps us moving, keeps the hope alive and the knowing that everything will be okay, even if it's not how we thought it would be? Read to the end of this to see what has truly pushed me to looking even deeper inside of myself.

On Friday my daughter Chaya Gittel (my only daughter, my biological baby who has Down syndrome) came home for the Sabbath. I had started to feel stronger, I could even hear my voice become less like a really old lady...well I'm sort of old...

At lunch on Saturday she had a seizure and has been in hospital with my husband...still not home! Tests show nothing and she is still to see the neurologist.

My amazing family rallied round, helping me with our youngest (not biological, also with Down syndrome). They visited the hospital and have been a huge support.

My strength in all of this after the last chemo came back – it just had to!! I thank God for helping me and for my wonderful family who I know I can rely on and love so very much.

APPROXIMATELY A YEAR BEFORE THIS SEIZURE, the house mother at that time at my daughter's apartment had informed us of her behavior. She explained that Chaya Gittel was in such a bad temper that she broke a school computer. We had not encountered this when she lived at home. Always a fun loving, happy girl, we were shocked to hear about this. They requested we attend a meeting, headed by a psychiatrist, to decide what to do.

Alarm bells went off in my head. A psychiatrist! Why? I couldn't understand why after one incident this was necessary. We later learned that it's part of the standard assessment process. I was convinced at the time, and maintained throughout every meeting, that Chaya Gittel does not have a behavior problem and it was out of character for her to break anything or to get up in the middle of the night and take blankets away from each girl, another incident they told us about.

At one meeting, the social worker attached to the apartment told us Chaya Gittel had for no reason stood excitedly and thrown something out the window. They never found what it was and I expected it was just her imagining throwing something out. The description of how her eyes were up in her head, and how she took time to calm down, alerted me to the possibility of her having had a seizure. The psychiatrist wanted to put her on medication. I was adamant and disagreed, insisting she should be monitored.

At a further meeting I asked for a reference for a neurologist, but the house mother was swamped with work and didn't make the appointment. Instead, halfway through, she was employed in a different apartment. Now we had to start again with a new house mother.

I resisted the need for medication for longer, but eventually we agreed after being called for several meetings. We were asked to check her eyes to diagnose her rapid eye movements. Chaya Gittel was taken by the house mother to a neurologist, who wanted to have her tested. We were delighted at the quick action of the new house mother. Before any of that could happen, the episode when she came home for the Sabbath took place. It was the end of the long journey and proof that she did not have a behavioral problem but was having episodes of disconnect. This is the latest term used for seizures.

August 3rd – FB post

I have physically been feeling so much stronger the past three days. Although I still feel nauseous every so often and I have a horrible taste in my mouth I actually want to eat now. I manage to eat tiny amounts but...I'm eating, which is the main thing.

A DEAR, caring, kind, wonderful friend recently sent me an email from someone she had subscribed to on my behalf, which helped no end. The information was invaluable. Some of it confirmed what I'm so blessed to have discovered and realized a while ago. Things like looking after yourself, following your gut. One of the things I found extremely helpful was to internalize that this is my body. I want to take back the power that I have handed to the professionals, for I instinctively know what is needed. I do not need to blindly follow but to ask questions, get curious, and follow my own common sense.

Common sense. I used to say from time to time, "He's really clever but he's not got any common sense." But what IS common sense? It is sense that is common to everyone – if it's common then it's known to all and therefore available to all, even if we don't know we have it. In my experience it comes with a feeling of 'oh yeah, I knew that' or 'of course'. It's so obvious, but maybe we couldn't see it before. Maybe another way of talking about common sense is calling it wisdom or insight. For me it often shows itself when I am calm, although it is not a prerequisite.

Ultimately what it meant was that I could rest easy in the knowledge that no matter what, I would know what to do in a situation. Now sometimes I might need information which will help me, but the answer will always be deep inside of me.

August 8th – FB post

Don't you just hate those (hospital) gowns you have to put on backwards? I always feel they would work better the other way round. Usually they have no ties or at very least they have one but nothing to attach it to lol.

This evening I will be donning this evening wear along with little blue booties for my bare feet. Yup time for another MRI...last time was shoulder, this time breasts to see if titanium wire is in right place and to use as a baseline...hmmm!

Fascinating information. Shaved hair side just itches loads. Hair on unshaved side at first was itchy. Now it feels like...well you know how sometimes you sleep and your hair goes against the direction? It's sore to touch and loads coming out today when I touch my head.

I'm in a place of loving and enjoying whatever each

moment brings. Definitely ready for the drilling noise of the
MRI tonight.

August 14th – FB post

Well here we go...2nd round of chemo.

Gosh, what can happen in a short time? Incredible!!

My sister is visiting me which has been such fun. We
have laughed and cried but it's so good to be with her. Love
her sooooo much.

I now have the result of the second part of my biopsy. I
have hit the jackpot! I am HER2 positive and although this is
an aggressive cancer, they have treatment which is hugely
successful...so sorry guys but I am going to be around for a lot
longer lol.

Finally shaved the rest of my hair as the pain on the
longer side was unnecessary. Most anyway has fallen out but
the process was hair raising.

Now here is a confession that not many people know. I
LOVE feathers. I have no idea why or when it started but I
just love feathers. I love to feel feathers and get them and
then take them from the stiffer hard bit and break them
down. I love to feel the feathers in my pillow and duvet.
There are often mangled feathers around me, depending on
my mood.

We bought some feather cushions for our garden to
brighten up the benches. I scattered them to create a lived-
in feeling. I heard rain was on the way so I brought some of
them inside. None of us contemplated the weather
changing so soon so I left some out.

Cars in Israel are often so dusty that the first rain only
dirties them. After the rain, I knew some of my beautiful

cushions would be wet and dirty. I carefully took the covers off the cushions ready for the washing machine. One of the cushions looked like it had already started to smell and needed to be washed as well. The others were fine once left out in the sunshine and shaken out.

Just before my sister arrived, I put them in the washing machine. The cushion, the cushion covers and, as I had plenty of room, some sheets and duvet covers from our bed at the same time. I'm a cushion, duvet and pillow washing expert. This was partly due to one of my children wetting herself regularly even with a diaper on. I was completely and absolutely astonished when Frank saw there was a problem with the washing machine. It would not open and there appeared to be feathers floating freely inside.

No problem. Just put it through a spin cycle and then into the tumble dryer and any small number of feathers would be taken off. No way! We ended up having to call a washing machine technician to help take most of the feathers out from the filter. As for the feathers, well, Frank filled up quite a few bags of the stuff and they did not come off easily. I am reminded of this each time now when I take out something like a pair of tights and notice a feather sticking in them. You just have to laugh.

When my sister arrived, she helped Frank to try and rid us of the remnants of the feathers in some of the duvet and pillow cases. They went outside to shake them. I couldn't help but laugh at the absurdity of feathers flying everywhere.

August 22nd – FB post

Sunday was such an unusual day!! Yes I know it's Tuesday, but my best excuse is that I have cancer brain. Yup, it's a real thing, and I'm sticking to it at the moment for my lapses in whatever.

First my son was leaving home to go to assisted living for the first time. He was excited and wanted his sister to see his new home. I was tearful...my baby was leaving home and I wasn't feeling strong enough to go with him.

My daughter has been asking when her next birthday is since her last one. She finally wore her house mother down and they made her a before birthday, birthday party. The girls in her apartment all travelled to our home to celebrate her 'fake' birthday.

MY SISTER HELPED plan the party. When I spoke to my daughter before she came, her voice was full of excitement. I love it that such simple things please my two youngest children. Everything remains as it was when they were much younger. The simple things in life are so thrilling for them.

All the girls from her apartment traveled to our home on the bus, a treat in itself for them. There was excitement and fun in the air. We invited friends that know her who live locally and some who were here on holiday to come and be part of the merriment.

The girls were all beside themselves with the food, the balloons, the guests. They played games. I managed to muster some energy. Out of nowhere and through not wanting to show my daughter that I didn't have the stamina, came a surge of adrenalin. And then just as suddenly as they arrived, they left, and I fell onto the recliner in a heap.

August 24th – FB Post

Just arrived home from taking my sister to airport. She came two weeks ago to help and look after me.

We had a few days of going out and about. Went to the time elevator where we saw history come to life in a simulator. Got bounced around a lot and couldn't stop laughing. Went out to see how cider, stout and lemonade are made at a cider factory called Busters (well it only had 5% alcohol). Then she came to help with my #3 son when I went for my last treatment. She sat there giving me the ice.

She has cajoled me, encouraged me to eat and to take short walks. We held hands to cross the roads like little old ladies – ummm I mean 'older' ladies. She sat next to me while I dozed off in my chair (OK – I admit – I snored!!). She brought me small pots of nuts and raisins and made sure I was drinking. She soaked prunes for me to drink the juice. She was there with me, just being there was such a comfort.

We laughed about old times and cried too. We took selfies with grimaces and just spent time being together.

Thank you, Amanda. I love you to bits. See you in October.

DURING AMANDA'S visit we arranged for an old friend, Devorah, to give us both a manicure and pedicure. I had never had a pedicure before. That's a whole new experience: having my feet shaved of all the old skin and painting my toe nails. We spent a couple of hours during the process, the three of us sitting, laughing and joking as if nothing was wrong, nothing had happened. An ordinary day.

I remember as a child, my mother coming to me all smiles.

"Would you like an egg?"

"No!" I would reply, annoyed at the suggestion.

Her face would drop for a second and then, when she had another idea to try and tempt me, she would smile widely and say, "Would you like...?"

I drove her mad refusing to eat anything she suggested. My sister reminded me of those days as she too would come up to me and say, "Would you like....?", only I just couldn't face many of her ideas.

At this stage of the treatment, although the pink stuff coursing through my veins was unpleasant, I was able to go out during the second and third week. The treatment week exhausted me.

I had a chronic cough. It started before I was diagnosed but I was sure the chemo was not helping. It persisted and eventually we called the local doctor. The nurse at the doctor's surgery was amazing. Unfortunately, my usual doctor was on holiday, but I saw someone else who I had heard only good things about. I literally walked in and walked out. Incredibly, there was no one in the waiting room as they had ensured it was empty and I wouldn't need to be near any germs. My immune system was low so I had to avoid sick people.

The doctor examined me, asked questions and sent me for an X-ray. So, off we went for the X-ray, which was then emailed immediately to the doctor. The silence was deafening. No one phoned to advise us what to do or what was wrong. Finally, we called the surgery, who told us they had sent all the information to my oncologist at the hospital. He was also going away that day but we managed to get him to look and send back word.

"It's not cancer on the lungs. There's nothing they can see on your chest."

What is it then? It didn't get better and I'd had it for over four months. It aggravated my throat and sometimes I wanted to be sick with the constant coughing. My chest hurt from all the extra work it was doing and it was sometimes painful to breathe. I needed to have it addressed and get to the bottom of it all. Now I had to wait until the oncologist returned.

FOUR
SEPTEMBER 2017

September 1st – FB post

Gosh I'm feeling as if I didn't sleep last night.

Yesterday the lovely Raizel came to visit and we did a Facebook live. When she left, I just needed to rest...even the smallest thing and I feel tired.

Anyway, I went to bed early but was woken by my husband's computer that clearly wanted to have a late-night party. I'm telling you these machines have a mind of their own. It seemed like I just finally dropped off again and there was a phone call for us to tell us that the transport for our son to take him to school would arrive soon...ummmm...he doesn't live here anymore!!

Then a second call from the transport for our daughter who moved two years ago. Well it was the first day of school, September 1st, and they are very efficient, lol.

Am still coughing my guts up but have my third chemo on Monday, so will hopefully get to see the oncologist who hopefully has returned from his holiday. My eyes feel incredibly dry all the time, unsure why.

Has a smell ever reminded you of a person or place? It has for me. I can smell chemo and biopsy and MRI rooms of ice and pink infusions and I can't get it out of my nostrils. I had a smell stuck up my nose many years ago about a holiday in Switzerland that I went on with Valerie and Helen but that smell was yummy. Just saying!

Now I always thought that being fatigued was for very old ladies (please not the VERY old bit). Sort of a word I associated with the 1920s when people didn't get tired but fatigued...yup I thought it was just a posh way of saying tired. But I keep hearing this word...so this is the word of the day and in context it means: I feel nearly dead from fatigue, figuratively speaking of course...coz I'm not dead or nearly dead – just not raring to go at this moment. zzzzzzzzzz

I MET Raizel in 2013 at a Three Principles conference held annually in London. She sat next to someone I had been working online with and asked if she knew anyone at the conference who might have traveled from Israel. She then sought me out and we have stayed in touch ever since.

Helen and I have been friends since we were eleven. We met in senior school and although we lost touch at one point, we found each other again. We went on a couple of school trips with my cousins Phillip and Valerie. I recall the thin chips they would serve us for our evening meal and the hot chocolate always available when we returned from the piste. They were heady fun days that I love to recall. The smell of that hotel combined with the smell of snow and hot chocolate reminds me of good, happy days of my youth.

September 4th – FB post

Here we go again. Once more into the unknown and feeling vulnerable. Round 3 of chemo.

I got to see the oncologist, who sent me down for an X-ray. Yes, another one. My eldest son had offered to come with me (as do all my boys) for this treatment. Once done and over with we returned to see the oncologist, who decided it was time for me to see a pulmonary expert.

I'm glad that something is being done with my cough. Every time I go for treatment I cough incessantly. It looks like during treatment my cough is worse. It's beginning to hurt my chest and I keep getting stares from people, perhaps frightened for their health with a sick person in the oncology ward. It keeps me awake at night too.

September 8th – FB post

Today is one of the worst days I have had since starting this blooming chemo stuff!!

There I was thinking that I feel okay...not great...but okay...and then whoosh! I feel more sick than usual. I cry for no reason. I feel weaker. I feel like...well like rubbish. AND I'm not scared to feel this way.

It stinks and if you're counting maybe this can be rant #2 (so who is counting?) but here's the thing...they told me that I would only feel awful for two or three days. They LIED. Ok maybe that's a bit strong...they told me things that I have not experienced!!

They told me the pills would stop me from feeling sick. All I would like is to swallow properly and stop feeling like vomiting. I would like the awful taste in my mouth to disappear and for the smell (even after the Vick under my nose trick) to leave and stop tricking me into believing for a second or two that I am in that room full of chemo drugs. I would like to walk without holding on to the wall for safety and to sleep without waking several times a night.

And then I look at the wall in my lounge where I hung family photographs. My parents are there, our wedding, my children growing up, getting married. My grandchildren (the light of my life) and I know that the way I feel is only temporary and it will go...and – I'm fine even though sometimes it doesn't look that way. Thank you for life...for my life!

SOMETIMES WE WAKE up and forget the gift of being alive. I have sometimes dragged myself out of bed and gone about my day without realizing what is around me. Maybe when we receive traumatic news, a shock diagnosis, we start to be more aware of our surroundings. I noticed though that being grateful for the little things around me started some time ago, before my cancer diagnosis.

In some of my darkest moments I heard something from deep within myself that shook me up and transformed my life from one of anger, frustration and unhappiness to being peaceful and calm, and to appreciating life with whatever comes my way.

I was lucky to have been guided to the realization that even when life looks like it sucks and is hard to bear, within that there are moments of peace and happiness.

I am reminded of the young man who came to visit me about five years ago. He walked in with an agenda, wanting to see something that would enable him to find his soul partner and finally be happy. His shoulders were hunched and he sat on the edge of his seat when he first sat down. From his pocket he took out a few sheets of A4 lined paper.

From the short distance away, I could see that his writing was scratchy, small and covered every inch of each sheet.

He offered them to me. I smiled and explained that I didn't need to see them. He carefully folded them up many times and pushed them into his inside pocket. As we spoke, he relaxed, sat back in the arm chair. His shoulders didn't sit next to his ears now and he looked younger. Suddenly he lurched forward, took out the papers, opened them and held them out in my direction.

He repeated this behavior a couple of times for the next hour, when he asked to use the bathroom. He walked tall and straight and when he returned he said, "I looked in the mirror in the bathroom and it was like a breath of fresh air. Life is truly wonderful."

He was so fixated with the bad parts of his life that he admitted he had forgotten to smell the roses. He kept beating himself up, telling himself there was something wrong because he was having recurring thoughts that appeared from nowhere. He thought he was useless and would remain single forever. All that happened was a shift in his perspective. A realization that no matter what goes on, he is still okay inside, even when he feels awful. We are built with a mechanism which aligns us when we go off course. Once we interfere and try to correct it, it keeps us out of alignment.

I knew that no matter what, this young man was perfectly healthy inside. I had every faith that he would find a partner when the time was right and if he didn't then that too would be alright. His happiness was not dependent on finding someone to make him happy. That's an inside job.

Needless to say, he wrote to me within two months telling me he was getting married to the girl of his dreams. He said that he woke up every morning and looked around, to smell, listen, touch and be aware of what was. Even the mornings when he felt less inclined to jump so quickly out of bed, he remembered that just like the clouds in the sky, our thoughts never stay in one place for ever.

September 13th – FB post

Today is a new day!!

I woke up this morning feeling so much better. I found a little bit more of my voice too.

I can feel when my white blood cells take a plunge. It's the little reminders like my eyes feeling like they have ten tons on each eyelash. That horrid feeling when you think you are starting to get cystitis and it's a little painful...eeeekkk.

BUT I am extremely grateful that I have my eyelashes and some of my eyebrows (and even more grateful for the stuff I can paint on them so no one knows their real status). I am grateful for the fact that I woke up this morning to be here at this moment.

I am more than grateful for my husband who is always so patient and kind to me. For my caring children who before I can blink, offer their help. I am grateful for my caring loving daughters-in-law who help brighten my day with their pictures, their WhatsApp messages. I'm grateful for my grandchildren who are the sweetest most caring little people...when they call me, my heart literally melts.

I love to tell this to people because it is so impactful. My daughter, who many would not call 'normal' (she has Down syndrome – and by the way, when I told her she has Down syndrome she said, "Ach, it's not important"), sometimes says to me when I'm clearly not present, "Mummy, where are you in your head?" I am grateful for that normality, that under-

standing at such a deep level and that love that my family gives to me on a daily basis.

I INVITE YOU TO START. Look at the light, start with loving yourself and see that light shining brightly inside you. It's always there.

September 17th – FB post

Have a cough. Been with me since before I was diagnosed with breast cancer. Has been driving me mad... cough... cough... cough. Nurse told me to see my doctor. But my usual doctor was away on holiday. Still went and she suggested I get an X-ray and then proceeded to pass me on to oncologist who was just about to go on holiday.

This sounds like one of those old-fashioned sagas or a soap on TV lol... And then dum dum dum dum

At last chemo two weeks ago I told the nurse that I never saw a doctor for my cough, and immediately found myself on another floor for another X-ray and then in to see oncologist who promptly sent me to see a pulmonary whatever.

Today, finally had the appointment. Now need to sit in a box and breathe for one test. Another blood test and a few other bits and pieces to try and get to the bottom of this cough.

The silver lining – coz there is always one. I have finally got a license for medical marijuana. From the country set to storm the world and send it out to all nations. It only took five weeks to be approved...and a further three weeks to wait for my 'dealer' to speak to me. Waiting!!!

Told you! Definitely a soap – and the best bit – it's in color.

September 19th – FB post

Yesterday was a crazy day. Woke up early and spent a long time in and out of the bathroom.

Got too weak and knew I needed to get some fluids inside me. My daughter-in-law arranged for someone to bring in something that would help but I couldn't drink it.

In the end my son came to drive me to a local clinic to get the fluids I needed. I walked in like a 90-year-old and walked out...well I could say like a 20-year-old but truth is walked out like me, a 62-year-old feeling physically so much better.

Was interesting that there was a point when I just intrinsically knew I needed to get myself seen to. Thank God for telling me when and what to do.

I'm always so fascinated that there is a time when we just know what we need to do. It's like, duh, this is obvious. Sometimes

the chatter in my head is so compelling that I get busy making up stories and scenarios instead of reading the messages about how to go forward.

September 24th – FB post

Early start tomorrow...4th chemo and last of the sucking ice one (I hope). The four treatments after this one will be chemo with targeted biological something or other.

Feeling pretty good going into this. Mentally doing really well. The old body might have something to say about the physical side of things but hey, as long as my head is in the right place, the rest will follow...ummmm where's those legs? Well I went for a walk with my head, just left the rest behind.

Got to sit in some sort of box tomorrow so I can do a lung test for the coughing thingy. Had a blood test today to test for whooping cough...well ya never know! Still need to do a test for TB...has to be something me thinks, but a bit of a mistake if it's none of them and I'm still coughing.

So tomorrow marks the halfway mark.

Still waiting for my dealer to call me with my supply of medical marijuana lol.

ONE OF MY SONS, Yosef, came with me today and Alister met us there. During the treatment the people from the cannabis depot called to say that I should go to a different hospital to collect my license and get my cannabis.

Yosef was delighted and although we had little time to spare, he drove me. We arrived at the hospital and asked directions.

"You see that ramp, go up there, turn left then right then straight."

We followed the instructions to a tee and arrived somewhere, but clearly not the medical marijuana department. We asked again.

"To the end, turn left then right, that's it."

We arrived at a completely different department and asked again.

"Turn left, go to the end then turn right."

We arrived and were invited to wait for someone to give me my 'stuff' and instructions on how to take it.

Can you believe, you have to have a lesson on what to do? For example, I had no idea that I needed to use a plastic spoon rather than a metal one to put the drops on. Then I had to slowly increase the intake, one drop at a time daily, once at night, once in the morning. The aim was to build it up to take away the pain and use tablets as well as drops. It's a whole new world out there.

This year the festival of Succoth is in October. We build an outside shelter which reminds us of the time we wandered through the desert. For us it means family time too and for everyone to move in with us. Our married children live about a thirty-five minute journey from our home and don't have the facility to build a Succah (which is the booth we use).

It is a busy time of year but my energies were low and I was due to have treatment during the seven-day festival. I knew I needed help with all the preparations and my daughters-in-law came in to help in one way or another. For me there is nothing more satisfying than seeing my family gathered around, having fun, laughing, sharing, playing games and being there for each other.

FIVE
OCTOBER 2017

October 15th – FB post

They've all gone. All my children and my grandchildren. They

have left and the silence is deafening. In the silence I realize something.

You see I worked hard all my life but it was always striving to get somewhere. I have been a teacher, then an advocate for parents with children with special needs, and more recently...very loosely speaking a 'coach'. Always in the helping field, but I got a kick out of it and then I wanted more of that kick and more and more.

Today I sit here knowing that since just over four months ago, my whole life has changed. My body has taken a huge beating with the last four sessions of chemotherapy and there are four more to go. However, I just see more and more that the love my grandchildren give me unconditionally, the support, help and love my children, their wives, my husband, my sister and my family give me is almost too much to know what to do with it but just soak it up and be grateful. I have no words for some of the things they do for me.

One small thing. I lost my hair...even up my nose!!! But please! Do I really still have to shave my legs? ...lol

Tomorrow is my fifth chemo. Out of my comfort zone again, a new treatment with different drugs than the four before and I have no idea how it will affect me. What keeps me going is love and gratitude and knowing that I do NOT control anything...it is what it is. Glad to be alive.

STRANGE THING, hair. The lack of it initially was shocking until I started to see how beautiful the shape of my head is. It felt strangely freeing. I was down to the basics and it showed me another way of seeing my body as just the vessel for my soul, my core, my essence. The hair will come and go but what's inside will always be there in its entirety and purity.

October 15th – FB post

Okay this has got to be the most annoying doo da ever!!! Me innocently asking one of the nurses about the pill I am meant to take this evening and tomorrow morning.

"Can you please tell me what Telfast will do for me? It says it's for hay fever...why do I need to take it?"

"It hopefully will prevent any allergic reaction to the Taxol. You have to come twice this week."

Thanks to this nurse who always has time to answer my questions and help me with everything...not much thanks to others who did not tell me.

This is particularly interesting to work out the logistics for us as I will now have to go tomorrow for the biological

treatment and then Tuesday for the Taxol. Crazy situa-
tion...my husband has to have a procedure on Tuesday and
one of my sons is already taking him. Now need to ask one of
the others to take me as my husband can't. Hmmmmm and I
have no idea when I need to go back on Tuesday.

WHAT ALWAYS INTERESTS me is that what seems like
a problem and maybe insurmountable somehow works out
the way it's meant to be in the end.

October 19th – FB post

My 5th chemo turned out to be in two parts. One on Monday
and the second part on Tuesday. Why? Because the first one
of the targeted biological treatments is given separately for
that time only. I'm guessing if you don't fall on your knees
and die then you are up for it next time.

The first part took five hours and the second lot took six
hours. It hurt when they allowed a faster flow into my veins
but if they hadn't made them faster, I would have had to have
taken my toothbrush and teddy with me.

They told me in two days I would start to feel the pain
and I should immediately start to take the very strong
painkillers they had set me up with. I had other ideas, now
armed with my medical marijuana...heh heh!!

Today is the second day and it knocked me for six. I
cannot believe the intense pain that is constant in my legs
and feet, let alone the tingling in my feet and sometimes my
hands. It's a pounding heavy pain but gets less intense
depending on what I'm doing...funny that, isn't it?....ouch.

. . .

HAVING the actual treatment wasn't too bad; it was the after effects that were a shock. Elliot and Goldie arranged to come with me on the Tuesday. It was a last minute arrangement as my husband couldn't be with me as he had to be in a different hospital. Now we had another problem. How was I going to get to the hospital without making my son leave his wife and three children to stay overnight and drive me in the next day? That just didn't sit well with me. In the end, a kind angel let me know that she was available to drive me.

In the hospital, my son asked about the length of the treatment. The bag looked big and I had no idea. He came up with this idea that we should count the drips going into the container before going through the tubes and into my arm. We counted drips per minute. He then Googled for a conversion and discovered it would take about five hours.

After being there from 8 a.m. waiting for the blood results to come back and the five hours of treatment we would not be due out until about 3 or 4 p.m. That's a loooong day.

October 21st – FB post

Ended up blacking out...now in hospital. Feeling much better.

IT WAS SATURDAY, the Sabbath. We had no guests, just my son Yosef and his girlfriend Ariella, and she is really part of the family. I felt very weak all day and in a lot of pain. The advice given to me by the medical marijuana people was to take three drops when I started to feel the pain. I suspect that by taking that and taking a strong painkiller I felt even weaker. I was later told that the cannabis could make me feel weak.

I went to the bathroom, feeling very shaky. I was not sure I could actually get up and leave the bathroom and it took all my physical effort. I just wanted to lie on the cool tiles and sleep. I slowly managed to get my body out of there. As I came out I was very aware of needing to sit – NOW. I managed to sit on one of the steps to the side of the bathroom. My husband and my son's girlfriend were the first people I saw as I came to. I had slowly moved backwards on to the stairs and blacked out. My son called the ambulance.

I wasn't quite with it and there were a whole load of men all around me. First they put me on the floor. Then they started taking my pulse and putting cushions under my head. The head of the local department lives behind us and he came in. He wasn't aware before then that I was having chemo. He was more than kind but firm when giving instructions to everyone around him. A cannula was inserted and a drip set up ready to transport me to the hospital.

My two eldest sons, Elliot and Alister, arrived not long after I was settled into a cubicle waiting to see a doctor. I observed their faces. They looked dour. Maybe they knew something I didn't. But then within minutes after Yosef arrived, the mood shifted and they started talking at a rate I could hardly keep up with. They were discussing a new wallet that Elliot had bought. They discussed its shape and size, perfect to fit in a pocket. Then the conversation moved on to board games.

My sons are avid board game players and spend time together to indulge their passion quite regularly. I'm not talking about the usual family board games that most of us were brought up with, but some very strategic ones, others based on luck and others a mixture of both. Either way it was serious business to them.

I was amazed at the lightness in the room and laughed afterwards when Goldie told me that Elliot had mentioned his concern at whether this was now going to be a common occurrence – me ending up in hospital for different reasons. Maybe the thought, which had also crossed my mind, was that a lot of people don't die of cancer but things related to it, like getting pneumonia and not being able to shake it off. I still had a cough and that played quietly in the back of my mind, then the thought would disappear.

October 23rd – FB post

Yesterday was a hard day. Well maybe that's not entirely true...some of yesterday was hard.

I cried when I was taken to hospital and saw my three older boys come visit. I cried at seeing how serious it all looked and how helpless I felt. But then I laughed when they started talking about the board games they play and the wallet which takes all their stuff without slipping down inside their pocket. I cried when they helped me walk to the car. This is not something I had planned for my old age...I wanted to die in my sleep, gracefully and quietly.

This cancer thing has brought me to my knees at times and I cried yesterday when one of my sons took me to an appointment and held my hand so I could walk. I would really have been happy to lay down and die. You see this time my bones ache from my hips down my legs to my feet and it is relentless aching, non-stop...tingling in my hands and feet too...and even my tongue. Hmm maybe that's telling me to stop talking too much!

But then I saw the small glimpses of different things. My son's girlfriend getting me a change of clothes in case. Her thoughtfulness in going out to buy me cream for my dry skin, slippers and lip salve. My daughter-in-law always sending me cool pictures of my grandchildren and both of them always asking what they can do for me.

Today I realize that it's all just one step at a time. There is no race. No time, nowhere to go, nothing to do. I will go up and down and some of my thoughts are awful, but not all. Even in the darkest moment I see a glimpse of something funny or heartwarming...something that tells me it's all okay...and it is.

I SUGGESTED I would skip the pulmonary doctor's appointment. I was exhausted from the ordeal the day before, but Yosef insisted I go. Frank had missed so much work with his own procedure and coming backward and forward with me that Yosef had arranged to take time off to take me. He cared for me. Held my hand as I shuffled through the hospital to the appointment. It was challenging for me to walk and took every ounce of my strength, but I felt supported. I had to lean on him, not only for physical support.

SIX

NOVEMBER 2017

November 5th – FB post

Still on the merry go round...

It's really strange not feeling the soles of my feet when I walk and my finger tips are all numb. Best bit is that my sister (who flew over to be with me again) and my dear husband have been making sure I am well looked after; my nail polish lasts a lot longer lol.

Tomorrow I go back again for chemo #6. Last chemo seemed to have lost most of my eyebrows so painting them in has been fun...one side goes up over my bone and the other underneath...lopsided face! Flying high though with the medical marijuana so who cares.

The steroids aren't helping my weight. Yup, it's gone up making me feel very uncomfortable. Going into this session though knowing I am so close to the end of this phase. After tomorrow there are only two chemo treatments left before my operation.

November 7th – FB post

We never know what will happen and we are not in control.

Yesterday was my 6th chemo treatment, only two to go and I was already feeling like I had this all sussed out. Come on, admit it, you might have thought the same!! Yes, I knew the pain would be really something else but I felt at least a little prepared.

Then I told the oncology nurse about the blackout. Things changed while I was listening. The puzzle pieces I had arranged no longer went into the place I had placed them and they were all jumbled up.

Treatment yesterday lasted from 8 a.m. until we got out around 3 p.m. That includes time for blood tests, waiting for results and for the drugs to be signed off.

It was a heavy day. I had steroids and the two drugs which I will continue with for a year AND the bone pain drug (targeted biological treatment). Now though they decided to split the targeted one into nine. Nine treatments, so one every week. My end of treatment of this phase will now extend until January 1.

I plan and then each time I am brought back and realize I am just not in control and this is best for me at the moment. I trust this with all my heart.

THE ONCOLOGIST SOUGHT me out in the ward during treatment. He told me that no matter what, he was there for me. Professor Cherny stressed the importance of telling him everything that I am going through because he cannot help me with things I don't share with him. He decided to reduce the intensity of the treatment and give it weekly instead of the huge dose every three weeks. Once again I felt reassured and loved.

Our 'dealer's driver gave us a call. He informed us that he would be arriving in about seven minutes. My husband grabbed the money to pay him and of course my license for the cannabis and waited patiently outside. Seven minutes passed and turned into twenty, and no sign of the driver. He phoned again to inform us that he was stuck up the road and he couldn't find a way down. We might have to go to him.

I started flapping because today was the second day after the lower dosage of Taxol. Thankfully the pain is less intense at the moment than last time, but it is still there. I can't move too well and I started complaining. My mind started to fill up with what I considered the injustice of the situation.

"How can he expect me to go up to get the marijuana if I can't move? And if he can't get here how can I get there? We pay for him to deliver rather than go and collect the supply. I'm not going to pay him if he can't be bothered to get down here somehow."

I started pacing a little and the pain stopped me short. That dull ache in my legs and knees going down to my feet and toes, tingling. I caught myself making up something that might not happen, and then next call was, "I'm outside."

Oh wow...I went there again. How funny is that? I started to react and jump down the rabbit hole. Sometimes I see it really quickly and other times I miss it until it is long past.

I noticed last time and this time that my fingers are looking pruney after treatment. The ends of my fingers, the paddy bit at the top, are all wrinkled. I look older than my

years. You know how sometimes you have been doing loads
of washing up or been soaking in the bath for too long? Fat
chance, ha!

The pain in my legs goes up and down and is pulsing on
my bones. It is unrelenting, growing inside of me, traveling
wherever it wants non-stop. Sometimes the pain is more
intense and I want to try and judge if and when I need to
take some more marijuana. I am aware that my voice always
sounds weak and shaky when I am in intense pain and the
treatment is taking its toll on my body.

The phone rang. It hasn't rung too often since my diagnosis. People prefer to either email or send a message via
Facebook or WhatsApp. Maybe people think it's easier for
me to respond in my own time. The house phone is on the
kitchen wall. Sometimes even the small walk from the
lounge is too exhausting. I'm not very stable; my legs often
feel as if they will buckle at the knees.

Frank came to tell me the name of the woman on the
phone. I slowly got up and made my way toward the
kitchen.

"Hi. How are you? How's all the family?"

I answered carefully, not knowing quite if the speaker
had heard about my diagnosis and called to ask me or if it
was just a general call. It's the same woman who called
me all those years ago asking if I knew anyone that might
be interested in taking home a child with Down
syndrome. His parents didn't want to look after him. I
wasn't sure about this call, so I wanted to listen carefully
before speaking. I guess my apprehension came out in my
voice. I was cautious, waiting to see which way the wind
would blow.

"You sound very weak, without energy," she suddenly
exclaimed.

"Wellllll, I have breast cancer and I'm not feeling too wonderful at the moment."

She continued, "Oh I had a small procedure many years ago like that. Now the reason I'm calling is because..."

My mind was racing. In one breath she changed the subject as if I had said nothing to her. Had she heard me? Is it simply that people don't understand, so not their fault? Is it that they just don't want to be reminded of their own experience? Or maybe they just don't know what to say? I found it odd but interesting.

She continued speaking, giving me names of people, most of whom I don't know. This one is married to that one and she and they and we and them. She weaved a story with people and places that she thought would impact me. Her tale started to turn and I sensed she was asking if I would consider a suggestion.

"She asked me if I could ask you whether you would be interested or know anyone that would take the baby with Down syndrome. I told her it must be twenty years since she took the last child..."

I was frankly going in and out of the conversation. I couldn't believe that I was being asked to have another child with Down syndrome, not just because I'm so much older but for goodness sake...I have cancer!!! I have no strength to look after myself well, let alone a baby!!

I reminded her that it was sixteen years since we took the unwanted baby home to bring him up with our family. I was still slightly shocked by the conversation and asked why the parents didn't want the baby.

"The mother doesn't think she can cope. She has other children to consider and she wouldn't have the time to see to this one."

"Please tell the mother, she doesn't know if she can or

can't until she tries. She has just had a baby. It's a baby who needs her help like all babies, at least try."

I was getting tired and wanted the conversation to be over. We ended amicably but I was aghast at the dismissal of my news and the insistence in asking her questions. She asked me if I would visit her as she now lives in an old age home not too far from where we live.

I left the conversation initially feeling annoyed with her but then gained an insight. In her mind she had a task to do; that was her goal, so anything I might have said outside of that framework didn't penetrate and it was easier to get her job done quickly rather than start to pay attention to anything else. She perhaps thought that her reply to my reason for being weak was enough. On the other hand, I have no idea what she was thinking at the time. How can I ever know what someone else might be thinking?

I did not know the pain would be so intense. I was hopeful for a full recovery because even though they had extended the number of treatments, they lowered the dose. The medicine coursed through my body and was at times excruciating. I wanted to rub it all away, but when I tried to rub hard, my bones and their insides felt raw. It was almost like I had no skin to protect me. The more I thought about it, the stronger the pain became. It never went away but was more of a dull ache, punctuated by sharp intense pain several times a day.

I am in pain but not suffering. Pain comes from my body, my outside shell. Suffering is something we experience from within. The pain is what it is but suffering is from me; I cause my suffering when I constantly overthink and then tell myself there is something wrong with me, which leads me to go round on the same spot. Stuck.

Suffering happens when I feel my own thinking and

then buy into its illusion, because I'm not suffering. I'm experiencing some bone pains, but my thinking about it can expand when I decide it looks so important that I must take note of it. It's a bit like a concertina: it opens and closes, and this can be done incrementally or with large sweeping motions. The suffering can end up looking like it's the very fabric of who we are, but it isn't. How can it be when I can change in a second?

Funnily enough I feel as though I have woken up from a dream. I feel more alive and more appreciative of each and every moment. I am grateful for waking up once more. I am starting to see more clearly what I really want to do. I have a vision, which was always quite cloudy, and I felt as though I was winging it before now.

It seems like the sides of my mouth are thick. There is a funny, strange taste. It has taken over and is constantly there. This horrid, metallic taste. Sometimes it's difficult to swallow. I have to admit that on occasion my mind has wandered to what it might feel like to suffocate, and then I shake my head back to reality. Back to the here and now. To the present moment. There is no time other than now, and what I have now is everything I need. It is only when I start to wander into past or future or start to think about the I and Me that I am taken away from this moment and into the illusion that there is somewhere else to get to.

November 12th – FB post

Woo hoo!! Finally bone pain in legs, hips, feet...all gone. Ready for treatment tomorrow. Should only be there for about five hours, but an early start again.

I could say that knowing the pain lasts from Wednesday to Saturday means I know what to expect. That is totally

untrue as I have no idea what it will feel like until I am in it
at that moment.

So here's to...whatever comes my way.

HAD AN EARLY START TODAY. Showered, put on
eyeliner and checked out the old eyebrows. Thankfully,
they still looked good. Am determined now to eat differently. Finally, I do not feel sick all the time so I want to plan
instead of eating for the sake of it...I prepared some grapes
and satsumas as well as a tuna salad for myself. Frank
would take pot luck with sandwiches the volunteers kindly
provide for patients and their carers. I was ready. Well, sort
of ready.

From early this morning, at about 6 a.m., my stomach
was complaining about yesterday's lunch. I had only eaten a
salad with sweet potato but for some reason it didn't agree
with my insides. I spent a while in the toilet and my mind
started to wander. What happens when we can't get to a
treatment? But then it all went out the window as I felt a
little better.

The treatment today was shorter and less painful. I
noticed my dry, pruney hands. I felt the liquid course
through my body, even to my insides where I was now
getting worried I might need to dash to the toilet. I began to
believe that I would be unable to make it and would make a
fool of myself, but then the intense cramping and pain
subsided and I relaxed. My fingers swelled.

We were back at home by 1 p.m. – another one done.

On the third day, I woke to gingerly use the bathroom.
My legs felt red hot to the touch. They're painful and
walking feels difficult. They feel like they are unattached to
my body. I am shaky and I know I have the stuff firmly in

my body. I just imagine Bambi walking with his very young shaky legs and it reminds me of my own.

We never know what will happen, what we will experience, and how we will react. I was beginning to feel stronger, wanting and even excited to do things. But today my legs are like pieces of cotton wool and my insides are like jelly. Weakness has set in and I am unable to stand for long or move too much.

November 17th – FB post

You really have to laugh!

I have two mosquito bites on my forehead. I mean come on mozzy what were you thinking? This blood ain't so good at the moment and on my forehead...Really?

Went to put on my eyebrows and I flicked my hair out of the way. Ummmm looks like you are on same level as that mosquito...you ain't got hair to flick.

This week was different from the other two treatments of this Taxol stuff. I have felt extremely weak to the extent that my legs have buckled as I walk. BUT the pain is less intense. Two days after treatment my legs were burning hot and it was painful to touch them...I mean the bones inside were, still are, painful.

I am so grateful for being able to laugh at all the small stuff and see that in between all the physical pain there are more and more glimpses of those beautiful moments.

NOVEMBER 20th

I went for treatment today. Just Taxol. The bone numbing treatment that makes my feet tingle as it enters my body.

We used to have a boy come to our house every week for the Sabbath. He came even if my boys didn't come. I can't tell you how he treated us: with such respect. I felt like a queen. I consider him like one of my sons. He gave me a ride to the hospital so I could give my husband time to work. It takes a toll on someone, coming week in week out every week and giving up your time, especially during work hours. We met my eldest son there, who stayed with me and drove me home.

On the way, my husband WhatsApped me. "Are you okay?" he asked.

"No, I'm dead."

After a short time he replied, "I've arranged the funeral. Do you want me to send a car or will you make your own way there?"

As quick as a flash I wrote back, "Depends on what car it is."

In response, his last message was, "Not much in the Save to Spend Pot and not appropriate to take it from the Fun Pot. I'll see what Avis has available."

Something that has helped us a lot in life is an online financial course. It changed how we spend and save, and how much we have for retirement.

As a result of the course, we set up different pots or spaces where we put our money each month. We have money earmarked as Save to Spend, maybe for a holiday or something else we want that we can save toward. We have a Growth Pot, which we use for our spiritual, intellectual and physical growth. We also have a Fun Pot for restaurants and family outings. This is all apart from a Giving Pot, where we put aside charity. A Necessity Pot is where all the things we need are earmarked, including food, gas, electricity, water, mortgage and other daily needs. Lastly, there is the

Investment Pot, which is where we put our investment money to compound and grow for retirement.

November 21st – FB post

Just got back from the local emergency center. Needed some fluids to bring me up to some sort of speed. Thankfully, now feeling a little better. They couldn't find vein in my arm so did it in my wrist...ouch not fun.

Yesterday was yet another weekly chemo. This time was really interesting as I could feel my hands and feet go numb as the chemo was going in. Even more scary was the fact that my tongue felt numb. Maybe it is a sign to tell me to stop talking so much, lol.

I'm tired and need to rest. I'm much more in touch with my body so I know when I need fluids, when I need to rest, or sleep.

MY WRIST WAS STILL HURTING this morning from the pain of the needle. So close to my bone. I wonder if I can wear my watch today. Or at least, on that arm. I had been a bit peeved with the doctor who inserted the cannula. I considered them to be inferior to the amazing people in the oncology department who never bruised or hurt when taking blood and setting up a cannula in my vein. They could always find a point of entry in my arm. Yet here in this clinic I considered them to be less able, maybe less professional. That was really unfair.

I judged him for no reason. The phlebotomist in the hospital or at a doctor's surgery is experienced in that field. They don't need to hook up the drip or administer drugs. In the circumstance I found myself, in an emergency clinic, the doctors and nurses are dealing with broken bones, taking blood samples, assessing injuries, reading X-rays and determining the casualty.

I was exhausted from the last few hours. I went to bed and spoke to my sister, who said something that changed my perspective yet again. I complained about the pain in my wrist. I told her they couldn't find a place so had to use a vein lower down.

"Don't forget, you were dehydrated."

My mind whirled. I could feel the cogs in the old grey matter churn. I put two and two together. If I'm dehydrated, it's difficult to find a vein. Oh dear! I judged and made my own opinion, not based on anything except my limited thinking. Now I had new information, the whole picture looked different.

NOVEMBER 24th

In just a couple of days, my eldest son will be thirty. I can't believe how time has flown and how grown up and self-sufficient he is. He has a wife and three gorgeous children. He has been working in a company for the last couple of years and received regular promotions for his unrelenting dedication and hard work.

Friday, Alister and Yosef were at home with us. They laughed and giggled nonstop while playing their board games. Both Alister, also a man with a wife and two children, and Yosef found their jokes hilarious. They plotted to wrap the present we had all bought for Elliot but hide it to tease him. In the meantime, they wrapped one of the children's puzzles we have stashed away in a toy cupboard for the birthday boy. To top it all, they wrote on the envelope of the card, 'Happy 40th'. This amused them for some time and all I could do was watch and enjoy the moment.

The amount of laughing and giggling took me back to when they were young, their carefree childhood. They would play and laugh, but when they did fight they remained best friends afterwards. Long after I had tried to get them to be friends and say sorry, they figured it all out themselves. They understood that the best thing for all was to get on with life and let go of grudges. This made me see that it is still possible, no matter what and when. This is something I have seen recently but so wish I was able to glimpse and appreciate when they were younger.

By profession I'm a teacher of physical education. My love for athletics drove me to want to share it with children. I was not clever but what they called a plodder. I worked hard and when I put my mind to it, I got good results. Before I applied for teacher training college, the British government decided they needed more teachers. They set up a marketing plan to bring people in and I got caught up in that crowd. That meant a lot of the people attending college wanted to become teachers for the money, not that the pay was so wonderful, and for job security. After my three years of training, the government decided they didn't need so many teachers after all and so there I was, passionate about teaching and unemployed.

I initially took on something part time in the same town in the south of England. After a few years, with little prospect of finding anything permanent, I left the profession to work in my father's business.

Fast forward several years and I was married and had my two eldest boys: Elliot, who was rising five, and Alister, who was two. It was time to return to work, but the only thing I knew how to do was to teach; I had no other qualifications or experience other than teaching. So I checked out several possibilities, but being a physical education teacher would mean taking time during evenings and weekends to arrange and referee at different sports venues. I did not want that and found a conversion course to become a junior school teacher. No extra curricula activities, maybe some books to mark: this seemed a more suitable profession for someone with a young family.

Ultimately, I was offered a job at a school that did not require evening and weekend hours to teach physical education. It was perfect for me. At that school I met three delightful young unmarried teachers, Devorah, Ruthy and Chanelle. Over the years we have kept in touch on and off, but many things have passed and both Ruthy and Chanelle live in the U.S.A. and are married, as is Devorah, who is more local. All of them have their own families.

Ruthy's mother called Frank to tell him that her daughter would be in Israel for a Bar Mitzvah and wanted to visit me. Because Ruthy was coming, Devorah decided to bring some of her children and they all came to visit. This was very special for me. I was moved that they found time in their busy schedule to pay me a visit. We sat and laughed and reminisced about the old days and other teachers and pupils that we fondly remembered. I am grateful to them for brightening up my day.

How many times do we jump in the shower, sometimes before the water has warmed up? Rush in, wash quickly, out, dry, dress. Maybe we have an appointment to get to, or work or even a school car pool we need to do. It's a weekday morning and we are in a rush, unable to spend the time for ourselves or anything but the matters in hand that need doing.

I recently showered and really appreciated the warm

water on my body. It's one of life's luxuries. I loved the water flowing like rivers over my skin and onto the floor of the shower cubicle and then down the drain. I felt it on my body, gently, slowly running away. Something so simple, not only taking a leisurely shower but being alive enough to really appreciate a commodity so precious.

November 28th – FB post

Where to start?

Sunday, my daughter-in-law made a surprise birthday party for my eldest son. Can't quite believe he's thirty. What a lovely evening and so nice to get out. My son hugged me before we left and for some reason I started to cry. I have no idea why, the moment of realization that I am really old. Maybe the thought struck me that this might be the last of his birthdays I will see, or maybe I was just tired.

Yesterday, Monday, was a very long day. We left home at 7 a.m. and didn't arrive home until about 7:30 p.m. First stop was chemo. My son took me to the treatment and another son met us there. Suddenly a woman started having what sounded like a panic attack. I started to cry, no idea why, maybe I was worried it could happen to me, maybe I cried for her.

Had about an hour and a half before seeing the breast surgeon about operation etc. so went to visit my daughter-in-law. Came back and I cried again. No idea if it was because I was happy or relieved or just felt the moment and a heavy load being released. This is what I heard. "I can't feel the tumor...either it's gone or shrunk so small or is fragmented but I can't feel it." ...WOW WOW WOW such amazing news.

It's a difficult time of year for my husband. He is an

accountant and January 31st is a major UK tax deadline. Giving him time to be able to do his work just made sense. I was exhausted for many reasons.

We had the usual wait for blood test and results to return. I noticed one woman was told that her blood test had come back and the result meant she could not have chemo. Instead, they eventually brought her two enormous bags of iron. Gosh, I'm sure with all that inside her she will make it to the moon and back.

Each time we have chemo, the oncologist has to sign off on the drugs. When eventually mine came, I asked why I only had a small amount. I knew that this particular week was what I called my big week: with everything all given at once I should have at least three bags of different medication. Frieda, my lovely nurse, who is always cheerful and more than helpful, told me she would check.

"I don't think the professor can count. He is brilliant but he got mixed up with my dates."

Frieda laughed but came back after a while to tell me that he had ordered the rest of the meds and they would show up soon.

During the treatment, Alister and Yosef, who had accompanied me, started talking about their board games and the cost of each one. My head was fit to bursting. Apart from that, my stomach was really bad, a side effect of the lovely chemo I was getting. In the end, for some peace and quiet, I sent them to eat downstairs. On their return, the conversation changed slightly. Now Yosef told me about his lunch. He had ordered sweet potato ravioli and was offered a sauce. He was horrified that the sauce was just the soup on the side.

I hope I never have to experience what I heard that day on the oncology ward. I heard someone start to breathe very heavily. It sounded like she was choking or having a panic attack. The breathing was loud and heavy, and people were moving very quickly towards her. She was out of my direct sight, for which I am grateful, but the room went silent. It was calm. No one panicked; we just sat there quietly contemplating, knowing that it could have been any of us. I held my breath.

I'm not sure if it was from fear for her and whether she was okay or fear that it could happen to me, but I started to cry. I have no idea what I was thinking and the truth is it doesn't matter. What I felt, though, was a moment of despair, as if dying was just all part of cancer and here it was presenting itself to me. Was it a sign? But then what sign? Then I felt this warmth come over me and concern for the woman's husband and all the nurses who must see all sorts of things on that open ward.

After what seemed like ages, with people keeping their conversations really quiet, some of the nurses moved away. The heavy breathing subsided and things returned to normal, whatever that is.

At the appointments with the breast surgeon he explains everything, even if I ask him the same thing over and over.

"I need to examine you. Please take off your shirt and bra and lie on this bed. Tell me when you're ready."

He came in from behind the curtain. He gently put my arms above my head and said, "I'm going to examine your left breast first, even though I know the cancer is in your right breast."

He was quick and thorough and asked me, "Can you feel the tumor?"

I shook my head, but was terrified that I had been mistaken so I had never voiced this to anyone. I had checked myself only recently and to my great surprise could not feel any lump. Was I dreaming?

"Neither can I," he said.

The doctor took time to explain and draw a diagram to show what this all meant. I was almost too scared to believe that I might not have cancer anymore, or at least that the tumor had miraculously gone. I hadn't finished all the chemo yet! I needed to focus on what was being said, needed to concentrate on the important bits to be able to go back and tell my husband. I felt that I needed to react like a responsible adult, but there was this tiny thing inside me that was getting excited about what this all meant. I didn't want to get too excited, as who knows what can happen?

It's now the day after the good news. I feel very strange, as if I'm a fraud. I no longer have a tumor, or so it appears, and yet I am still going through everything I went through before this revelation. Now I am not sure if I dare say to anyone that I'm in pain or that I still need chemo. A friend came yesterday and she was surprised that I couldn't just stop all the chemo. She asked why I still needed an operation, and why I would even need to continue with any more treatment if there was longer a tumor.

It seems that the treatment has been accumulating. Whereas the leg pains used to kick in two days after treatment, now it's constant. It comes almost immediately as I am sitting there feeling the liquid trickle into my arm. A sensation comes over me, one of, 'Oh, here it goes again'. It's that feeling of loss of control. It's this warmth that comes from deep within, a knowing that although this feels horrid physically, I'm still all there mentally.

My eyes are really dry. I remember being told that it is as a result of the cannabis. So funny: my face, my skin feels so soft. Then I realize it's because my fingers are constantly numb, so everything feels soft.

Goldie had arranged for Elliot's surprise birthday party to be held at her parents' home. Luckily it was local, but we had to be there early before Elliot arrived. I was tired and feeling very weak so was not sure how quickly I could get myself into action. At one stage I was not sure if I would make it, but I pushed myself in honor of the day. Goldie arranged for someone to draw caricatures of people there, which was fun. Our picture hangs on my wall and in true caricature style gives me a big grin on my face. It makes me smile each time I look at it.

SEVEN

DECEMBER 2017

December 5th – FB post

One more bites the dust...only four more of the evil, silent, magic potion to go.

I committed at the start of my cancer journey to be honest and upfront about my treatment and everything that goes with it... So, here goes for some more truths.

Neither the breast surgeon nor I can feel the tumor. Brilliant, wonderful news...and then the guilt sets in as well as the thought that I'm a fraud.

Guilt because maybe I no longer have cancer so I got away with something (no proof of this, but still, it came into my mind). I'm a fraud because I'm going for treatment, need an operation and radiotherapy and people do not understand why any of this is needed now. Yup, some people think I just need to stop it all and just get back to my old life.

I would love nothing more than to get back physically to at least how I was before my diagnosis. However, the lessons I have learned have been invaluable, and although I would not wish this on anyone, I have had the biggest wakeup call and insights into what life is about.

Tomorrow I have an appointment for genetic counseling and a blood test to see if it's hereditary. Becoming a little difficult to find a vein lately.

MY RIGHT ARM has decided it prefers not to give blood. I have been advised to give it a couple of weeks before trying on that arm again. Not a big deal, just a nuisance to only have one working arm.

DECEMBER 6th

Today, finally, is the appointment for the BRCA test. First, Frank and I had to have genetic counselling. We were taken into a small room and asked about our family history. The likelihood of my cancer being genetic is very low, but the answer is needed to decide what sort of operation I will need. If the results are positive then I will have a double mastectomy, but if not, then a lumpectomy will be enough.

After the history lesson, I needed to have a blood test. So, armed with a small plastic bag with some vials and a paper, we made our way down one floor. The blood test left my arm with a bruise. Next stop was to pay for the blood test so that we could get the results back within a week. If we had opted for the local clinic to sort out the same blood test, it could on average take two to three months. At the end we made another appointment for the following week.

So now I am very busy socially, with three appointments next week. Of course, there is the usual chemo treatment on Monday, MRI on Tuesday evening and then the results of the BRCA test on Wednesday.

My skin has become scaly and rough. There's a long patch on the outside of my arm between the crook of the elbow and the elbow itself. The information available says that rashes are a side effect and I had pills to take to alleviate that. However, as there was no sign of problems earlier, they told me to stop the pills.

December 11th – FB post

One less after this morning's treatment. Only three of the Taxol to go. The Taxol is the one that has been quietly sneaking into my body and giving me all sorts of interesting symptoms. Heh heh! Nearly got you beat even though you have tried to beat my body up.

The drive to the hospital today was just breathtaking. I saw the most beautiful colors in front of me. The leaves of the trees were turning from green to burnt orange and some even to a bright yellow in the midst of the dark green leaves that still remained. Even the trees with no leaves stood there majestically.

You know, it's interesting. I don't need to do anything to tell the trees or plants what to do and how to shed their leaves or whatever they need to do. How incredible is life. Nature just knows what, when and how.

EVERY TIME we go to the hospital there are no disabled parking bays free. I reckon that all the people with disabled badges park there the night before. Then they go home by taxi and return in the morning for their appointment and leave at some stage with their cars. Either way, it is a miracle to find a space, and yet today there were three spaces. What a beautiful day this is.

It seems that the vein in my right arm is really in need of a rest. The 'blood lady' said I should wait a couple of weeks before we try using the veins in that arm again. My arm burns when the Taxol goes in so it has to be dripped slowly. After waiting three hours until nearly 11 a.m. for the treatment to start, it meant that a good part of the day would be gone before we could leave.

After the treatment, sitting here at home, I feel okay. The small things that keep occurring have become almost the norm now. My nose is constantly sore inside. I put Vaseline in my nose each night, but in the morning when I blow my nose it bleeds. Two days ago, I noticed that my arm has become itchy and sore. It looks like I have eczema and it has worsened. It's just another symptom from the drugs inside my body.

The inside of my mouth feels thick. That sounds a bit weird but to be honest, it feels weird. It feels as if my cheeks inside my mouth are thick and it makes my mouth feel smaller. It takes a while for my eyes to focus. It's like the edges of my eyes twitch all the time. The main thing though is not actually being able to see clearly for a while. I have got used to it and know that by the end of the day it will all have settled down.

I was woken up just before 4 a.m. with a stomach ache. It is normal to wake with the pain but not always so early. I was surprised, in particular because I had not eaten that much the day before. I hate this part of the response to my treatment. Sitting on the toilet is something I do most days, no matter what I eat.

December 12th – FB post

Well guess where I am tonight? Waiting for an MRI. Must remember which way round to put the gown.

Guess where I will be tomorrow morning? Getting results from my BRCA test.

Who says I don't have a rich social life?

THE NOISE WAS RELENTLESS, like a drilling sound and then high-pitched noises. Even with headphones and some classical music, the noise was deafening. The session thankfully only lasted thirty minutes.

December 13th – FB post

Finally, we have found something that shows I'm normal. BRCA test is normal. Woohoo!

So funny what excites me now...years ago it would be to see the look on my parents' faces when I wanted to walk bare foot in the street. Well I was a hardcore hippy lol.

Ok well back to the medical marijuana.

I COULD NOT BE MORE DELIGHTED at the news this morning. A weight is gone. My children can relax and I can have a lumpectomy, not a double mastectomy.

So funny what excites me now...years ago it would be to see the look on my parents' faces when I wanted to walk bare foot in the street. Well I was a hardcore hippy lol.

Okay well back to the medical marijuana.

December 14th – FB post

Life is like a roller coaster.

One of the things I have come to understand deeper and deeper is that I am not in control of absolutely anything in this world.

The results of the MRI our daughter had after some seizures were in. They suspect Moyamoya disease. This is degenerative.

Whoooosshhhhhh hold on, here we go again.

SHE HAS TENDED to have whatever is written in the book since birth; it was wishful thinking for it to be any other way. A rare degenerative disease, which without treatment is fatal. I am devastated.

A friend persuaded me to go out with a group of ladies to a local restaurant for lunch. I hoped to avoid any crowds but just wanted to see and be with people, in particular as hardly anyone visits. Tasting anything at the moment is not pleasant or exciting. I tend to go for foods like curry as they are strong and spicy and I can actually taste something. There was no such option and the food once again tasted bland, although the company made up for it.

On Sunday morning Joyce, a close friend, came to paint my face. She had been planning a birthday party for me in her home and part of it was to put makeup on. As I sat there it seemed so surreal to be having my face made up like a child who needs help. I felt helpless.

The room was full of ladies, balloons and a table packed with goodies. I was determined to try as much as possible. Each person brought a platter of something with them for

the occasion and I was asked to taste them all. Sadly, I
tasted nothing except too much salt, too dry, too sweet, too
filling. This might sound ungrateful and it was not meant
that way. I have little excitement at eating. I can fancy
eating something, get up, arrive at the fridge and decide I no
longer fancy it. Sometimes I take it out, heat it up and it just
does not taste how I thought it would.

Treatment on your birthday is not ideal. Joyce and her
sister-in-law Naomi wanted to join me for my treatment.
My husband drove us and we arrived in good time. Frieda,
my nurse, was not in the clinic and someone else was
assigned to me and took me under her wing.

Sitting waiting, not knowing if the blood tests are okay
to continue treatment, allows me time to rest and sometimes
have a nap. Today, though, the waiting was with friends.
Joyce brought some nail polish with her and painted my
nails. What a birthday treat! However, the time went
slowly, it dragged on seemingly forever, and it was not until
two and a half hours later that treatment was started.

This was the last of what I called the double whammy
treatment. I would have the daily weekly Taxol plus
Herceptin and Perjuta all on one day. I was prepared to be
at the hospital until late, but getting off to such a slow start
would make it even longer. In a way, I was hoping to be out
and home by about 4 p.m., at which time my children and
grandchildren would come to celebrate my birthday
with me.

Only one drug was brought out. The other drugs had
been forgotten, something which occurred last big
whammy day. What would happen if I didn't tell them?
Don't be ridiculous, this stuff is helping, just open your
mouth and tell them. Stacking things in your favor is always
a sensible route. The drugs were ordered, but the late start

meant that we didn't get home until nearly five in the afternoon.

I flopped down into my inviting rocking chair, flicked the bar on the side to raise my legs and then took a breath. I looked around the house at my grandchildren playing happily and realized that my family is just everything to me. The distinctive taste of fried fish, chips and tartar sauce tickled my taste buds and I ate something. Dessert was full of sweet delicacies which I would normally be a big fan of, but today my stomach was not interested.

December 22nd – FB post

Thank you to everyone who sent me birthday wishes. Really appreciated all the kind words :). I was thoroughly spoilt by friends and family.

Last week, on my birthday, we left home just before 7 a.m. and arrived home at about 5 p.m. after a long day of treatment. What a birthday treat to see my grandchildren and some of my children waiting for me when we got home.

One less of this horrid Taxol. Next one is Monday...ho ho ho...Xmas day. Last one of this drug is on New Year's day then full steam ahead for the op. More getting undressed, more gowns and deciding which way round to put them.

We had a wonderful weekend with all my children and grandchildren. My daughter unfortunately spent most of the time having seizures.

To all my friends who celebrate Xmas, have a wonderful day with all my love, xoxo.

MY NOSE FEELS MORE sore than usual. I cannot stop sneezing and blowing my nose. I have tried to avoid this but finally it caught up with me. I just want to do nothing and am even feeling sorry

for myself. I hate that feeling of being unable to breathe properly.

December 24th – FB post

Crying for joy...can't see anything on MRI...tumor might have disappeared.

THERE'S HOPE. Even in the dungeon of darkness, there's always a glimmer of light.

The surgeon once again explained and drew another diagram of the different scenarios that might have happened. Either there really is nothing, but they have to open me up to check, or the tumor is now in smaller particles around the area. Either way I hope that the operation won't take as long.

The lymph nodes are small round organs found in several places around the body. Lymph nodes are important parts of the body's immune system and they monitor for the presence of foreign substances, such as bacteria and viruses. If a foreign substance is detected, some of the cells will become activated. Lymph nodes are also important in helping to determine whether cancer cells have spread to other parts of the body.

The sentinel node is the first node where cancer might have spread.

The surgeon, in his soft quiet voice, explained the procedure. Nuclear dye will be inserted, which will show up during the operation and enable him to know which node is the sentinel node. This will then be sent to the pathology lab, and while he is waiting for the result the removal of the tumor will be completed. If the sentinel node shows up as cancerous he will remove other nodes that have been infected.

If more nodes than the sentinel nodes need to be removed, a drain will be inserted to take fluid away from the area. This will need to be monitored and, depending on the daily measurement, will be removed within a couple of days. There is a danger of lymphedema, a swelling of the tissues in my arm, if they have to take out nodes.

It started as a tingling; I wiggle my toes. It creeps upwards, the numb feeling, slowly taking hold. It continues up into my tongue until I can't feel anything. It becomes stronger, more definite, and my top palate becomes numb as the pain in my foot starts to throb without giving in. What is this new symptom?

December 27th – FB post

This week has been exhausting. Today was the third visit to the hospital.

I felt so ill this morning that we left later than hoping to and I didn't take my marijuana tablet. I cannot believe the pain in my legs from this evil Taxol. I am also very shivery and weak. Lesson learned: take marijuana.

Everything I try to eat tastes like metal. I have even tried chocolate and I never thought I would say it, but it tastes yuk.

Now if you think I have been winking at you...sorry, it's the muscles in my eyes twitching lol. I wouldn't mind but when people do visit (and they have been few and far between, because let's face it, just as when I had my daughter with Down syndrome, people think it's catching. It's only cancer. If you sit on my chair you won't get it...and no, not everyone dies of cancer and it is only a word, it does not define me or anyone else that happens to be going through or understands this experience)...people say I look good.

Just ONE more Taxol to go woo hoo!! Phase one nearly done.

DECEMBER 28th

I'm really excited. Amanda is coming to visit once more. Her flight is in the evening, so I have time to make sure I am well rested.

Plans made have a habit of being unmade. I hoped that the family would come home for the weekend to see their aunty but on Friday morning, Goldie called to tell me that Ari and Talia were not feeling well, and the doctor advised her against bringing them to be with me.

Meantime, Alister also called to tell us that Yocheved, their daughter, had a temperature. All a guess, as they used their hands rather than a thermometer. My sister, the nurse, gave them instructions. They came, although Yocheved had red eyes, but by the time she was bathed and had eaten, she looked much healthier.

Yosef came home early on Sunday evening. Frank was using the time my sister was with me to travel to London and do some work.

Orly, my niece, arrived Sunday afternoon and insisted we took a banner to hold up above our heads in Arrivals at the airport to mark her arrival. Amanda and I spent time in the morning cobbling together a couple of sheets of paper with some tassels made with brightly colored ribbons and a stick. We created a flag with her name on it written brightly and boldly. I was excited to see her but wished it wasn't under these circumstances. You mean you wished you were not ill?

EIGHT

January 1st

Early start. Off for the last of the Taxol. This drug has been hateful, with horrid effects on my body, and I will not be sad to see it go. I sincerely hope I will never see it again.

There was a big surprise when we got to the hospital. Goldie arrived with bagels and a cinnamon bun for all to share. A celebration. My last day of Taxol and hopefully on to the next phase. I could see the end of this horrid ordeal and it seemed that the worst was over with this last treatment. We sat and laughed, reminisced and talked about what we would all do when all this would be long forgotten.

My father's Yahrzeit (anniversary of his death) was on Tuesday, and to commemorate we met up with the family. I hoped I would be able to go to a restaurant and treat my family but I felt very unwell and weak, and had a really horrible taste in my mouth. Instead, they all came to our house and we ordered food to eat in.

The last of this batch of treatments were very difficult. Whereas earlier, I was able to come home and have at least that day and the next fairly free of too much pain, now it is constant and unforgiving. I came home ready to flop into a chair and do nothing. I couldn't eat and, although it was nice to have family around, I was in no fit state to have much of a conversation about anything with anyone.

Having my niece and sister visiting together was a treat. Although I felt weak, we sat and binge watched a show nearly all day for the few days we were together. I was moved that Orly left her three children and husband to visit me. The preparations for her children to get to and from school must have been enormous work and I will always appreciate her being with me.

During one conversation with one of her sons, Orly turned the phone to face me. Her son asked in all innocence, "Is Graunty Susan dead?" I must have looked a right fright to him. Orly's children call me 'Grauntie', a shortened version of great auntie.

January 7th – FB post

Belated Happy New Year to everyone. How exciting to know that this year might be very different from last year.

Today my daughter had her second MRI – we hope to have results next week in time for our neurologist appointment.

I finally finished that evil Taxol on 1st January 2018. This drug accumulated and my body took a beating and I'm still waiting for it to leave me. My sister, niece and #3 son were with me. I am more than grateful that my sister came again to spend time with me, look after me (even if she is a bit bossy lol) and that my niece was able to fly over too.

My husband flew to London. Jolly good job too. He can't be spoken to at the moment until the end of January as this is his busy time working on all his clients' accounts. Bear with a sore head, me thinks. Tomorrow is an easier day. Treatment is with Herceptin and Perjuta. Much less time as don't need to wait for blood test results, just a cannula and the poison. Waiting for operation date.

My husband's work takes him to London several times a year. For the most part I am happy to be left at home while he leaves on a Sunday afternoon and returns late Thursday evening. It used to be once a month, but of late he has not been travelling as frequently. He travels even less since my diagnosis.

January 9th – FB post

You know when you know something will have to happen but then you are told when...

Eeeekkkkk my operation is set for Sunday.

Have to be in hospital by 7 a.m. to have a hook put in my breast. The operation will be late in the afternoon, when they will inject me with some nuclear stuff and the surgeon will use a Geiger counter. Click click click, lol.

Apparently I will look grey after...a bit like death warmed up. They will open me up, take out a couple of lymph nodes and test them. In the meantime, the surgeon will make sure to take out anything hanging around in my breast (if there is anything). Test results on the nodes they take out will determine if they close me up or remove more nodes and insert a drain.

AT LEAST THIS time I have a better idea of what will happen. I know that if they have to take out the lymph nodes, there is no need to wake me, as they said when I had the cyst. I also know they will give me a lumpectomy and there is something to be said for not having the fear of possibly more comprehensive surgery such as a mastectomy.

I hadn't realized I would be called so quickly and told that it would all happen the following week. On the other hand, there was little time to think about it all before I had to go in.

January 14th – FB post

Had to be in hospital 7 a.m. 6th floor to ward...wasn't sure if I needed to go to general surgical or geriatrics lol.

After half an hour I was sent to the third floor to have wire put in my breast. No local anesthetic, was tongue biting. Then they gave me a mammogram which not only made me bite my tongue but inside of cheeks too, and my eyes went cross-eyed.

Back up to the sixth floor and given a bed. Soon need to go to fourth floor to have some nuclear medicine put in. Back up after to sixth floor then down to fourth floor to check there's enough dye in me.

You guessed it...back up to sixth floor until 2 p.m. when they will take me to second floor for operation. Giddy just thinking
about it.

January 14th – FB post

11 a.m.
Ouch ouch ouch ouch.
Four injections around nipple to put nuclear stuff in.

THE WHOLE DAY seemed like a dream. I wasn't sure

why I had to be in so early, but soon realized that waiting to go from one place to another and from test to test was the reason.

Apart from the operation taking out the tumor, that in my case had either broken down into small pieces so wasn't detected or had indeed vanished completely, they had to check the lymph nodes.

The injections around the nipple were fast, apart from the last one, which seemed to take much longer and stung more. The surgeon who was to do the operation did the procedure. It stung and there was no numbing cream applied.

January 15th – FB post

After having nuclear stuff put in I returned an hour later for them to check there was enough in the area. Big machine, three scans each five minutes long with time between for the machine to change angle. Quite painless but clearly my counting from 1 to 60 x 5 was out a bit.

Got ready for surgery at 2 p.m. yesterday (seems like it was ages ago). Went down to pre-theatre room and was transferred to a different bed in the theatre. Some show they must have seen; I knew nothing of the play at all after the injection.

That injection...well. "Just a small prick in your arm," followed by the most excruciating burning pain. "The burning is just the stuff going in... Good night Susan." Then I knew no more till they called me again to wake me in recovery room.

They found cancer in my lymph nodes so they were removed. Now walking around with a drain. Results will be back in about a month when they will know if they removed enough and I go back to see if I need further surgery and how much radiotherapy I need.

One more night in hospital. My lovely #3 son Yosef stayed in hospital with me last night. All my family were with me (not the little two with Downs, they thought I was going in to have a baby and thought it was most amusing).

January 22nd – FB post

The last few days have been hell. I have wanted to crawl into a hole and for it all to end. I wanted it to stop...the pain, the need to push myself to exercise with the pain. Cancer. Just stop!

Someone came to visit me Friday and I cried. I have cried every day since and I'm going to say what I said earlier...cancer stinks.

In between we had a diagnosis of Moyamoya confirmed for our daughter. I don't even know how to begin to thank Avital Chevern for her care and help throughout all of this.

Isn't it funny though, through all of this there are moments when I see things around me almost as if they are larger than life? Last night my husband went out to deliver food to one son and an umbrella to another. I put on music and I danced.

I DANCED around the room with a freedom, an abandonment full of love. I just wanted to be in tune with how my heart felt and I danced with tears in my eyes but brimming full of pure love.

The words just meant so much to me...*I hope You Dance*. What a wonderful song to dance to.

NINE

FEBRUARY 2018

February 12th – FB post

Have been slowly healing and doing my exercises. I am not quite able to raise my arm straight. The scar is still numb, so is my armpit and the underside of my arm. Went to see surgeon last week before he went on holiday. He was pleased with how the scar was healing.

Today was appointment with oncologist to hear when radiotherapy will start.

I am gutted...results back from operation show that they did not take enough out from my breast. I need another operation. This is just another blip and it is what it is but I was still surprised and disappointed. I cried when I heard the news but was comforted by my sister, who is visiting again, and she held my hand.

FRANK, Amanda and I went to the appointment to see the oncologist. I was full of hope and anticipation for a different outcome. It just goes to show that expectations are just that.

Some things we expect to happen, but more often than not, they don't.

Amanda left for London on Thursday afternoon. My brother arrived Saturday evening to spend a few days with me. It seemed like we were backward and forward to the airport lately. I was glad to get out the house and walk around.

FEBRUARY 19th

Pre-op again. I have to go through the whole system once more. I saw the nurse, who took notes while chatting to me. Then it was out to the waiting room, looking at the screen to see when I would be called again. The anesthetist was the same woman I saw on my original visit to this department. We walked into the room and she looked at me with disdain. I figured that her face was set for everyone with this look, as I remembered it from last time. I asked her, just as I had done previously, to speak to me in English. She refused. I was firm and insistent.

"Last time I was here you spoke to me in English so I know you understand me."

Stony silence.

"If you don't want to speak English then it is my right to ask for

someone to translate."

She sat, looked at me and then slowly started to speak to me in English. My brother was horrified. We laughed when we came out the room at the ridiculous situation, for no reason.

Finally, after an ECG and examination, we were free to leave. Next stop was to go to the breast health department to drop off the paperwork and see if they had a date for the second operation. I saw Susan the nurse. She hugged me and I promptly started to cry. I had had enough of being pushed and pulled from pillar to post, one appointment to another, with no time to breathe. It's rare to need a further operation, I was informed, and so my question was, "Why me?" Again.

FEBRUARY **20**th

My brother Anthony, who is eight years younger than me, left. We dropped him off at the airport and I cried. He's so kind, funny and helpful. I had so much thinking about him coming to visit me. He has called to speak to me periodically during the last few months. He told me he was coming to visit but it didn't happen and I felt angry that he hadn't made the effort to see me earlier.

I had forgotten about being in the moment. Being present with him meant that I realized in a deep way how we can all get blown off course, believing something is the right thing to do or be. We hold on to stuff, and yet there may be a different way to approach things, more kindly and gently. I held on to my upset, disappointment and anger and yet it all melted away when I was with him. We connected again and nothing else mattered.

Frank had a bad cold; actually, this was one of a few he's had this winter. I sent him to the doctor. I could not afford to be ill. Now my throat hurts and it has been days since I have been able to swallow properly. I started to cough and it got progressively worse. It was evident that this might not go away without some medication so I asked Frank to make me a doctor's appointment.

The doctor listened to my chest and looked down my throat and ears, and I started to cry. I am concerned because

I must be healthy enough for the second operation. The cough was hurting my chest and it was hard to breathe. It was too much; I wanted it all to stop. He prescribed both Frank and myself antibiotics, and within a couple of days the symptoms subsided.

I was feeling sorry for myself. I got down there and spent some time wallowing in self-pity, which did me no good at all. I felt it, let it walk through and out the other end, and leave. Those negative, self-pitying thoughts come and go, but from time to time I take them seriously.

February 25th – FB post

...I was told the numbness in my hands and feet may continue for up to two years.

Clearly, I have not undressed for enough people yet, lol. Back in to hospital this evening for my second operation tomorrow morning.

This will all end soon. I'm amazed at how calm I am and that I know it will all be as it is meant to be. I'm so glad that I'm not in control of any of it and I can just sit back and observe as it all happens.

FEBRUARY **26th**

I had to go into hospital the night before the operation so I would be assigned a bed. I had hoped to be able to walk in first thing in the morning, as I didn't need all the tests that were performed before the first operation.

When we arrived, I was told there were no beds on the surgical ward so I would be given a room in a different ward. We waited to be seen and finally I was shown to a room and my bed. At least I could eat and drink until midnight. I was the second on the list for the following morning. They estimated I would start at 10 a.m.

I lay on the very narrow bed and waited for them to put the arm stirrups in each side. First my left arm and then the right. The nurses, in the meantime, put the little discs around my chest to monitor my heart and then started to bandage my legs. I lay there while they put equipment around me and then told me I would feel a prick in my left hand. Once again it was painful and this time did not seem to go in the right place. The anesthetist slapped my hand and moved the needle as the pain seared through my hand and up my arm. I stared up at the two huge round lights above my head. I felt dizzy and then I was asleep. When I woke I was in the recovery room and so glad to be alive and out of the operating theatre.

My body feels as though it has been excavated. My chest and back are sore when touched, as if someone has been mining and now all that is left is an ache. The sharp pangs that come when I move in a certain direction, either stretching or reaching, are almost electric. My muscles feel as though they have seized up and are warm to the touch. I am not sure where to massage although I am sure that it would help. All I want right now is for my arm to get its full use back and to be able to move freely without needing to gingerly reach or maneuver to avoid any pain. I feel as if I have been punched in my chest and my back.

Just home from hospital yesterday and I'm tired and in a little pain. It's all sore again. To be honest, I am tearful; I feel as though I am in a nightmare which is taking too long to wake up from.

All I want is to get my strength up again and to be normal, whatever that is. I used to want to dig around and find the reason for the sadness, but I know that it doesn't matter why – it is not helpful to know the content of my thoughts. What is helpful is to know is that just like the weather they will go and something new will blow into my mind.

I would love to spend more time with my grandchildren, help my daughters-in-law so they can work freely without having to worry who will pick up the kids or sit with them when they are sick. I want to be able to get up and about and start to do a little more. I have felt so out of life sometimes, just being able to give in to the treatment. I was shocked at how my body couldn't do anything, and the only thing I could do once again was to sit and be.

I wanted so much to help my daughter when I thought she needed me. To my surprise but great pleasure, I saw that she was perfectly capable of adapting and working things out for herself. I believed that the medication she was taking was overkill. This was confirmed by the doctor we saw, who is an epilepsy specialist. I could see the tremor in my daughter's hand, how she switched her cup of water from her stronger left hand to her right, which was not shaking as much. I watched as she negotiated stairs and ramps and told me she could manage herself. I was proud of how capable she was, always prepared to try and do her best.

From the outside, I saw her persistence and the amazing way she just gets on with her life without complaining. She does the best she can all the time. Her inbuilt ability to work things out, to know what to do, is a shining example to us all. She might not be able to learn in a classroom as well as some others, but she is in tune with her wisdom, and trusts that to her core.

FEBRUARY **28**th

I'm glad to be home but feel the tears constantly. I am so grateful to be back but I am scared of the next results and whether they have finally got all the tumor out. My experience of all that has gone on in the last couple of months has been a much gentler ride than the one I used to be on. I feel a calm and a knowing that no matter what, it will be how it is meant to be. One of the things I have noticed on this journey into the unknown has been that I am not in control and that listening to my body, resting when I need to, is one of the most important things I obviously needed to learn.

My body is bruised and my arm is sore and painful. At times, even when I reach for something there is a shooting pain, as if an electric shock is passing through my body. I have been told that it's all the nerves knitting together. I trust that my body knows what to do to heal itself. The underneath of my arm, the armpit, gets stuck every so often to the side of my body and I have to carefully prise it apart. It's as though the skin gets attached to the wrong place and needs to be moved away gently.

My mouth is sore from where they put the pipe down to intubate me. I'm glad though that it doesn't feel as bad as last time. I can see that within even a day, it has started to heal.

I watched as we drove once again to the hospital, a follow-up appointment with the surgeon. I noticed the bent trees, trying to get out of the wind. I noticed the way they gently swayed in time with each other. They grouped together as if looking for warmth. I could almost hear the rustling of their leaves, dry and crackling. The silver of their bark and branches stood out and shone in the sun.

Even though they are bent and appear older than they are, they are strong. They continue to be a symbol of nature and how magnificent this world is. Their might and unwavering steadfastness give me strength. I am inspired by these gentle giants. Set back from the road, they look brittle, as if they might snap, but they just move to the music of the cold, wind and rain.

I have no idea why, but God wanted me to slow down, to take a back seat. I have had no option but to do so. I have had the chance to breathe the air, to observe life as it has flowed past me. The slowing down process took some time and I certainly tried to fight it initially. Why would I want to stop or even start to slow down? I was convinced that I needed to continue to help others and be a service to them. But what service could I be to anyone else, let alone myself, when I was resisting and fighting against all that was meant to be?

Although I doggedly continued with clients, my mind started to forget things. I was unable to focus for any length of time. Out of the blue it occurred to me not to coach 1:1 anymore. It doesn't feel right to me at this moment. I get so caught up with wanting people to hear the message that I think I am too forceful. I read an article not long ago about hearing the principles, and it doesn't mean that everyone has to go off and teach them, preach them. Surely it is more important to show by example, to live them?

I know that my outlook on life has changed. I see things differently now and I hope that somehow I manage to put the words onto paper and have some impact that way.

TEN

MARCH 2018

March 1ˢᵗ

Purim. This is a lesser-known Jewish festival in which Jews give gifts of food and drink to at least one other person, donate money to charity and listen to the story of Esther, often in synagogue. It is a time when people wear costumes, celebrate publicly and drink. It is really the only time that Jews have permission to drink alcohol freely.

Every year we invite whoever wants to come by to celebrate with us. Frank makes a huge BBQ and the drinks run freely. We have many boys, sometimes between forty and fifty, coming in and joining the fun. Some spend time sitting with us and some just drift in, have a drink, eat a little and leave. The music rocks the house and some stay and dance. Our children and grandchildren also come to be with us. It is lively.

At first, we were unsure whether we would open our home this year. Would I be up to it? But we decided to go ahead, and if necessary, I could go to my room.

I listened to the music as the boys started arriving and

bottles were opened. I had time to relax and just be. The music was loud but my mind was not busy with a million thoughts driving through it. I felt my whole body relax. There was a peace inside and an alignment, which just came together without me doing anything. I know in times past that listening to music has touched my soul; I enjoyed a freedom and aliveness inside that was peaceful and happy. What a wonderful day.

The day after Purim, Frank went into the center of town to the shops to get some things we had forgotten to buy for the Sabbath meals. When he returned he said, "I'm sorry, I have bad news for you. Helene died on Tuesday." I was devastated. Helene was the reason we came to live where we do. I suddenly saw how life goes by so quickly, and here but for the grace of God am I. In one second, we take our last breath and then we are in this physical world no more.

I was heartbroken, especially as only the other day I had thought of her and resolved to call her when I felt stronger. Now it will never happen, and although we didn't see each other often, she will always be in my heart and my thoughts. It's the finality of death, the end of being here. It's also the fear that maybe I am next. No matter what anyone can say, no one knows our destiny, no one knows when it will all end. I feel like I have done my work here, whatever that might mean, but who am I to know or understand what that entails?

Truth is, the moment my husband told me, I felt anger welling up inside me. I was hurt that no one had come and personally let us know sooner. I was in shock, but still the anger showed up and started to eat me up. I sent a message to my friend Sharon to see if she knew about Helene's death. I thought I would find out first if she had been informed and then ask why she hadn't told me. We exchanged messages and she called after to ask my forgiveness for not keeping me updated. She was trying to protect me, thinking that as I had not long ago had an operation I might not be up to hearing the news.

Initially I was upset with Helene's family. Why hadn't they called to let us know instead of Frank finding out almost as a 'by the way' part of a conversation when out shopping? Sharon reminded me that Helene's family are private people and it was a complete shock to them, totally unexpected. They were dealing with their own grief and loss. There I was thinking of myself instead of realizing this is not about me at all. Goodbye my dear friend, I wish I had been a better friend and been there for you more often.

Pain is part of life. We all at one point in our lives feel some sort of pain, whether it's from falling over and grazing our knees, breaking a leg or going through chemo. However, there is a difference between pain and suffering. Pain is just me having an experience of a part of life. I don't give it much credence, it just is. I am sure that it means I don't suffer, but take it all it my stride, so to speak. It's the feeling of being grateful that is helpful.

We tend to suffer when we mull over things, regurgitate the same old information or story and get in a frenzy about it all. The pain is not doing that to us. It can't, because we don't even experience pain unless we think about it, so it doesn't exist unless we have a thought about the pain. It is then that the continuous thoughts circulating in our heads create that suffering.

. . .

MARCH **14**th

Two days ago I went to see the surgeon. He was very pleased with his handiwork.

"Sit here on the bed and lift up your top. You don't need to undo your buttons. I need to see both breasts to compare them. It looks very good, kept its shape, just a bit smaller."

Tuesday is treatment day. Going every three weeks means I almost forget what it's like, but the smell keeps coming back in my nose a couple of days before I am due to go back in. It only takes about ninety minutes nowadays, so thankfully it's quick. Recently they decided they no longer need to take blood and now use the cannula only.

I can only use my left arm now for a cannula, to take blood or to have my blood pressure taken. They recommend I wear a sleeve and maybe a glove on my right hand, in particular if I fly, as the pressure in the cabin can cause swelling in my arm, but the final decision on that will be taken by the physiotherapist, when I am able to see her.

Any breaks in the skin on my right arm can cause complications and swelling of the arm. Things I wouldn't have considered are not endorsed, including having my cuticles cut or putting my hand or arm in very hot water.

Today I was determined to shop with Frank. I have not felt well enough to walk around and do a big weekly shop for the last eight months. The day after treatment it would have been impossible. But today was the day I wanted to go. The walking exhausted me and I felt weak. My legs ached and I collapsed into my chair when we returned, not wanting to move an inch. Then it hit me, the shivers and shakes, and I couldn't move, my energy was sapped.

There have been times when I have really wondered who I am. Am I the cancer that has taken over my body?

However, I'm not broken just because I have cancer; I am more than what my body has. From time to time I still make up who I think I am and start to feel sorry for myself at the terrible life I have and how awful all the treatment is. Then I know that I am so much more. I am still here, still breathing, still able to laugh and be serious. I happen to have had cancer. Apart from the physical pain and discomfort I have encountered, I don't really care that I have cancer. At first it was something I could use as a talking point, but it really doesn't bother me that I had cancer; it is not who I am.

I love this quote by Amir Karkouti, a Three Principles facilitator:

'The world wakes up with you when you wake up.'

My world only exists when I'm conscious, when I'm aware of it. Our consciousness helps us to be aware, to be able to see, hear, smell and bring in our senses, and to make sense of the world we live in. This might sound as if I am completely mad, but I'm able to feel each and every feeling with more aliveness than I ever did when I tried to suppress and be in fear of them. Being conscious and understanding that each feeling is just that, and is not telling me who I am, has allowed me to experience everything in full-on 3D multi-color, but at the same time to know that it's all okay, no matter what I'm feeling, and to be aware of and in the moment.

MARCH 16th

The other day I had a sore on the side of my mouth; today I have some on my tongue. My bones still ache and I feel at times as if I will faint. I had to sit several times at home and wash my face with water to keep me awake during the day. I was close to suggesting I go to get fluids, but I knew first I needed to sit and chill. I needed space for the feeling to pass, so I waited it out.

Someone on Facebook told me that their boyfriend's cancer has spread to his lungs and is growing quickly. I'm devastated at the news. Is it because the first thing I think about is me and question whether the same will happen to me? The next thought that comes through is "My gosh, you poor lady, my heart goes out to you". I want to help but words are all I have and they seem inadequate. What do you say to someone in this situation? I will be there for you...but I'm not and I'm not in a fit state to travel and help. Besides, what could I possibly do except be there for her while he is going through the pain? I am so sorry.

March 18th – FB post

I have some exciting news.

A few days ago, I put my hand on my head and it felt different. I took two fingers to my scalp, put them together and gently pulled. There is something to pull, a small amount of hair has started to sprout.

I'm still waiting for results from the second operation and until I get that I can't start radiation. They will come when they are ready and at the right time.

Last week I had treatment, at least it's only every three weeks now. Forgot what it was like. That smell as you walk in and the after effects. It knocks the stuffing out of me physically but I don't think I have ever been so okay as I am now emotionally, mentally.

March 28th – FB post

Some brilliant news! The second operation was a success. Next step is on to radiotherapy.

A surprise to be told I need to take a hormone pill for five years. Just when I thought I'd finished with the hot flashes and in this heat.

A NEW PHASE BEGINS.

April 5th – FB post

Yet another treatment completed.

I find I have no expectations of how it will be and am surprised when the liquid going in gives me a slight burning sensation. Did this happen last time? Did I feel so cold and shivery every other time? Did my bones really ache so much, did my joints hurt before?

Does it matter?

One less in a series of stories I could tell myself before and after.

THE NEXT MORNING, I woke in pain. The bones in my legs ache. The joints in my hands and legs are painful, stiff and difficult to move. Having expectations means that I believe something will happen in the future. How would I or could I predict what will be? When I let go of expectations, I'm not making up stories and convincing myself they will or have to happen.

April 10th – FB post

I'm not sure what to write first. All I know is, life is definitely not boring.

Went to hospital hoping to have my planning session for radiotherapy. Turns out it was just an exercise in note taking (again!) and being told I will need twenty-one therapy sessions. Was hoping at same time to collect my marijuana but turns out they only open on Monday.

Now next week will be exciting. My daughter has to go in for the final test to see whether she will need to stay on medication for the rest of her life or have an operation for the Moyamoya. She needs to be in Sunday morning for tests throughout the day then a procedure Monday morning. So there's a chance for me to collect my marijuana in between. Tuesday she'll be allowed back to her apartment.

Tuesday morning I will have a simulation of the radiotherapy (it's apparently not treatment, just going through it). I haven't been on a simulator since Disney in Florida...hope it's as exciting. Wonder if I can choose the tattoos they will put on my breast for the radio?

IN ACTUAL FACT it was nothing like a simulator but was a machine that works out where to put the marks on my body so that they show up when radiotherapy starts.

My first radiotherapy appointment. Just finding our way through the maze of corridors and rooms was a feat in itself. I was glad we had left early to allow for time to find the department. In my head it I thought this appointment meant an immediate start to radiotherapy and was a little disappointed that it was just to give me information. I hadn't realized that because this was a different hospital, I would need to register with a different oncologist for this part of the treatment. We were shown into a room where an intern waited. The young man proceeded to enter all my details into the computer.

Once that was complete, Dr. Sapir, the oncologist, came in and introduced himself. He looked at my notes, questioned the intern and then once again explained to me that I would need twenty-one sessions. I would be expected to attend every morning, Sunday to Thursday, at the same time each day. Once a week, on a Tuesday after treatment, a doctor would be available for me to meet so he could check the area where they were going to zap me.

A follow-up appointment was made for 17th April. The doctor explained that I would have to undergo a session where they would mark the area for treatment. The nature of the therapy prescribed was for sixteen general around the whole breast and five targeted specifically around the scar area and lymph nodes.

APRIL **15**th

Sari, the house mother where my daughter lives, has been reducing Chaya Gittel's medications, under the instructions of Dr. Eckstein, her neurologist. Now they are ready for her to have the angiogram that Professor Cohen suggested. I contacted Avital to see where to go next. Avital, in her efficient way, spoke to Professor Cohen's secretary and explained that I was waiting for radiotherapy. The secretary suggested they could do the procedure on Monday 16th April, but that Chaya Gittel would need to go into hospital for tests the day before.

Avital told the house mother about the need for Chaya Gittel to go into hospital from Sunday till Tuesday. She arranged for girls to take turns to stay with her in hospital throughout the day and overnight, which meant we were free to go home and get some sleep. Armed with the necessary paperwork, we met Avital, Chaya Gittel and Chaya, the girl who was to stay with her for the first shift. We went to register in the hospital and were sent to the neurological surgical ward.

Although Chaya Gittel is an adult in years, she is a child in many ways. The head of the ward recognized this and agreed to appoint her a bed immediately instead of waiting for the doctor to see her before admitting her. This meant that Chaya Gittel was able to get changed into hospital pjs and watch TV, much to her delight. She was kept amused for hours.

The day went slowly, with nurses coming in and out taking blood pressure, taking blood and checking her oxygen levels. She needed a chest X-ray, so we took her down to the X-ray department and Avital offered to accompany her into the room. With Avital's background I was delighted to have her with us. We had this feeling of being secure with the help all in place around us. I know this permeated from us to Chaya Gittel, who took everything in her stride.

Later in the afternoon Alister, Yael, Yocheved and Esti came to visit. Yocheved was delighted to sit next to Chaya Gittel and watch TV. It was a real treat for her. I couldn't resist and we put Esti on the bed too. The picture was perfect, all three of them goggle eyes on the TV, absolutely fascinated. Chaya Gittel, always the social butterfly, was so happy to see everyone.

From walking little and then going to the hospital, in that first day, I walked nearly 5000 steps — a huge amount for me. We left at 6:30 p.m. as I was exhausted. There is something about hanging around hospital that tires you.

We arrived before 8 a.m. Chaya Gittel had a good night, although she woke for a few hours. She had not had anything to drink or eat from 12 p.m. so we were hoping that she would be first on the list. Usually the procedure was done under a local anesthetic. We arranged for a general anesthetic as we knew Chaya Gittel couldn't stay still for long.

At 10:30 a.m. Chaya Gittel was taken for the proce-dure. Within an hour we were told she was in recovery. The procedure entailed putting a catheter with a camera attached through the artery in her groin, up through her heart and into her brain. The result of the test would help the professionals decide the next and best course of action for her.

On instructions from the doctor and nurses, Chaya Gittel had to keep her leg as still as possible for six hours after the procedure. At first, she had the wound strapped so her movement was limited. Keeping her leg still for six hours was not as difficult as we first thought. She was mesmerized by the television above her.

APRIL 17th

My appointment for the simulation in readiness for the radiotherapy was today. We managed to get to the hospital early to visit Chaya Gittel, who was pleased to see us. Our visit was short so I could go to my appointment in another part of the hospital. We waited outside a room clearly marked 'simulation room'. My mind wandered to the last time I was in a simulation, but that was many years ago in

Disney and was fun. Would I be jolted around in the same way?

I had to undress and lie on a table which moved toward the CT machine. The machine whizzed and whirred and took 3D pictures in preparation for the treatment. It worked its magic for fifteen minutes while I had my arms above my head, forbidden to move.

Out of the CT machine, they drew straight lines in the middle of my chest and from just under my collar bone to the bottom of my rib cage. The markers smelt, and when Frank and I went out for a walk later in the day, that's all I could smell. I noticed there were flies flying around me. I swatted them but they kept coming back. I remarked to Frank that maybe they could smell the markers, too.

April 23rd – FB post

Double whammy tomorrow. Morning at one hospital for first of 21 sessions of radiotherapy. Afternoon back at usual hospital for continuation of biological treatment.

What a busy life I lead.

Tiring week last week with my daughter in hospital for three days for her procedure. Now waiting for results. Thanks Avital, you are a saint. Will never know how to thank you.

APRIL **24**th

Chaya Gittel came out of hospital today. The results will come in on Monday after Professor Cohen confers with his peers.

On Monday, Avital called to let me know that the results would take another week. Professor Cohen was on holiday and although his secretary assured us there was nothing life threatening, this was upsetting. Yet another lesson showing me I'm not in control. I was saying how wonderful it would be to receive fast results.

———

IT IS A VERY EFFICIENT SERVICE. I was given a card to swipe on arrival and I received a ticket telling me which number in line I was. Frank and I traipsed down the corridor looking for room 38 and took a seat, waiting to be called. Large glass doors opened only when someone having treatment went in or out. I was waiting for them to position the machine, and for the computer to record it so that each day it was only seconds before treatment would start.

Once through the glass doors, I was greeted by such a sweet lady, who explained that I needed to put on the gown she gave me and then wait again to be called into the room. She informed me that I will have twenty sessions, which I queried as the doctor had told me twenty-one. Seems like I will need to speak to the doctor to confirm.

It was painless. Legs in one position, arms above my head, chin raised, not on my chest. The machine moved around me slowly and then stopped for a while before moving round to another position. I lit up when they used laser lights to align the position of my body with the lines on my body. I glanced up into the machine as it stopped nearly overhead. I couldn't see anything inside but there was an aperture which opened and closed from time to time, before moving round to my right and the side of my breast.

This visit was longer, as they needed to align every-thing, and now they drew feathers from the side of the lines. The smell lingered. Before leaving, they showed me where to place my gown ready for tomorrow, in a little cubby hole marked with my name and a bar code. I was sent down to the nurses' station for them to complete some notes on their computer. They spent time telling me about the side effects of the radiotherapy. I have some fun things to look forward to if they ever happen!

Tomorrow and for the next twenty sessions it will be an early start. My appointment is at 8:10 a.m. so I will need to be up early to shower and drive to the hospital on time. We left the hospital and drove home, had some lunch and then set off for Shaare Zedek for my usual infusion of Herceptin. We are hospital hopping.

I was ready for an early night. We arrived for my appointment on time the next morning but the nurses seemed intent on having their break before giving me treatment. Eventually I was called in and went to my cubby hole to retrieve my gown, but it was gone. Maybe I was looking in the wrong place.

The nurses invited me into the treatment room. They found it amusing that I couldn't find my gown and pointed to a chair and some food. I couldn't make it out. Was it a sandwich? I reached for one but it fell apart and they laughed. I woke with a start at 4:10 a.m.

That day my gown was taken and I was given something in the meantime to cover me sufficiently to walk from the changing rooms. I already knew it would be gone – I'd been given the heads up!

Throughout my time of treatment, when with friends and family and in replies to my posts on Facebook, I have often been told: keep fighting, be strong, you can beat this. I don't know how to be strong – what does that mean? I was told I'm courageous but I'm no more or less than anyone else, I just know all I need to do is put one foot in front of the other. It's all okay. It's just where I am at this moment. It doesn't define me. It makes sense to me to be. There is a deep sense of love and knowing that whatever will be will be.

I could be a millionaire if I would get one £/$ for every person who sent me a different way of eating, drinking, sleeping. I have been sent different diets, different alternative therapies, and all of them are interesting. Initially I looked through them, seeing what I could do to improve my health. I saw people making a fortune selling courses on eating in a certain style and swearing that it cured them from cancer. They told stories of how we have caused cancer because we don't know what to feed ourselves. But I realized that slowing down and being in silence was the answer for me. I was advised by some not to do chemotherapy, but that is their advice and is not coming from my wisdom.

May 4th – FB post

First sleep in this week...ahhhh! Had nine radiotherapy treat-
ments now. Feel very dizzy at times and starting to get very
tired after each session.

My energy levels have shot up since the chemo has left
my body. I am grateful for improvement each day.

My mind has slowed down since my diagnosis of breast
cancer. I have time to smell the roses, and they smell amaz-
ing! Lately with the burst of energy comes wanting to get
back to work...but then something gently taps me, reminds
me...living in harmony, with love and laughter, is more
important than trying to do anything. And so it flows and I
find I'm doing things that don't have that word work
attached to them, I'm having fun.

MAY **8**th

Today, as every day previously, we left at 7 a.m. and
arrived forty minutes later. If we leave ten minutes later, we

hit traffic and find few parking spaces, and could end up being late. Today, the computers were down and the machine which I have to swipe to register wasn't working. One of the technicians walked towards me and advised me to hold the card, which has a bar code on it, farther from the machine. Still not working.

"Don't worry. It says number five in the top corner so when they call that number you can go in."

The screen at the end of the corridor, outside the double doors into the treatment area, came up with 'room thirty-eight, ticket number eight, enter now'. That was strange. Is there something wrong with the machine? The next number came up on the screen so I decided to enter and let them know I didn't have a ticket. I was greeted by one of the technicians.

"Susan, get undressed immediately. Why are you waiting? Go now."

"Oh, sorry" I replied. "I was told my number was five so I didn't know it was my turn."

"It is your turn. Hurry up, get ready."

I quickly undressed and went into the room. It was 8:25 a.m. The same technician said to me, "You always come so early. You were here at 7:30 a.m. and now you are angry that you had to wait. Your appointment is at 8:10 a.m. If you come early then you will get angry at waiting."

I was taken by surprise at the force of her words. I explained quietly that I was most definitely not angry but confused. I got caught up in her words though, and lay on the bed feeling upset and attacked.

On leaving the room and getting dressed, it suddenly occurred to me that what I had seen was a lovely, kind lady who was struggling, trying to get on top of the list of people waiting as the result of the computer breakdown. It had nothing to do with me, although it jolly well looked that way for a few minutes. I laughed inside. We all live in separate realities.

May 14th – FB post

Sixteen down and five to go! The countdown starts.

First sixteen radiotherapy sessions, have felt very tired. Just takes over like a cloud enveloping me, I give in and sleep. Have to listen to my body. My skin is very dark and feels sore to touch. I often have sharp pains that shoot through my breast.

Last week went into the room with the simulator once again. This time along with the lines they drew at the beginning, they included a beautiful perfectly round circle. The last five sessions will zap that area.

Something new again. Going to a different treatment room. Infusion day as well tomorrow so long day out at two different hospitals for the treatments. Never mind, at least I got another batch of marijuana today.

Hard to believe that for the most part, the treatment is all but done.

THE SECOND ROUND of radiotherapy treatment used a similar machine to the first sessions. The round part of the machine that usually comes over my breast and to the side had an additional part attached to the end. It was almost like a square camera lens. It enables a more targeted way of treating the spot by the scar.

It was painful to lie on my left side with my right arm above my head. The skin around the scar stretched. It was difficult to keep it in the same position. I hoped it would end soon and then realized that the more I thought about the pain, the more painful it became. I relaxed and let the machine do its work.

MAY 15th

At the next Hadassah Hospital appointment we were early, so we decided to sit in the large foyer and people watch. On the way to the radiotherapy department a volunteer looked at me, smiled with a hint of pity and offered me a food package.

"Gosh, I must look like some old lady who is in need of sustenance to keep her going," I mentioned to Frank.

"You do look awful today."

Well thanks, I love you too! Are you meant to say that to me? I thought it was very funny.

As it was Tuesday I needed to see the doctor, so we waited outside the allotted room. She was inside, but then the door was flung open and she left. We waited ten minutes, then twenty. I needed to be at another hospital for my infusion, so Frank told the oncologist. Finally, she arrived, and once again I had to show my breast; at least this time it was a woman, although I have got past caring who sees my breasts.

Looking back at the time, it seems as though it's been weeks since starting the radiotherapy. I can't believe I'm nearly done with this treatment phase. I'm so tired, I want to crawl into bed and sleep for a week. Have to keep going.

May 16th – FB post

Seventeen down, four to go. I dragged myself out of bed this morning. My body is tired, my bones and joints ache.

But then the phone call came. "Suzanne," (that's how they pronounce my name here) "The machine is broken. It won't be working until about 11 a.m. You might not come for treatment today. If you do, we'll call you."

You know that feeling when you have it all planned, even when you don't realize you have it all planned in your head. Go for treatment, then shopping, rest and write some more for the book...Weeeeelllllll heck life is interesting, playing with me, gently nudging me to see that I'm not ever in charge.

So, still four to go.

MAY 18th

I broke a plate yesterday. It slipped from my hand and fell onto the work surface in the kitchen. Shards flew and a couple hit my wrist on my right hand. Knowing that infection is the enemy, I quickly cleaned it and put some antiseptic ointment on the affected area.

Frank and I went out to the shops. Entering the spice shop is an exciting outing, full of different smells and interesting pots of powders, some in glass jars. The jars are similar to ones I remember from my childhood that were full of sweets. Other powders are in large open baskets. The aroma was delectable and we walked around buying what we needed. On the way out, I slipped on a ramp. I fell backward and hit my wrists on the ground.

I could hear Frank shout out, "Oh no!"

I slowly sat up and took a moment to assess if or how much I had been hurt. My right wrist near the cut hurt and the vein was sticking out like the hump in pictures I'd seen of the Loch Ness Monster. We slowly walked home and drove to the doctor's surgery.

Observing people is intriguing. People assume you should feel and react in a certain way. I watched as all around me started to get into a mode of how they thought I should feel and how I must behave. It was quite alarming to see the vein sticking so prominently out of my wrist, but I wasn't frantic or overly concerned. I did feel weak and a tiredness came over me, but I recognized that as my body telling me I needed to rest a while so it could mend. Of course I would need to check it out, but I was not distressed by it; yet others seemed to play that role for me as if I should be down there with them.

MAY 22nd

Last time. It was my last radiotherapy treatment but the machine didn't register that I had an appointment. Apparently, the regime was changed and I finished yesterday. We waited for an hour to see the doctor and receive the discharge papers. I'm free. My heart sings and I cry inwardly with joy. I'm done! Another phase drops out of sight.

I have been blessed with the opportunity to reflect, to sit back and relax. To observe all around me. This time was a healing inside where my wisdom takes me, where it suggests and points to. Looking out each day at nature gives me that sense of wonderment that I had forgotten about in all my rush to live life according to my expectations. Stepping out of the busy world that surrounded me and I believed I needed to be part of has been freeing.

There have been many moments of sheer delight and a letting go of all that I thought was important. At times during chemotherapy, I was unable to do anything but do as my body bid. There was nothing important enough to worry about. There was nothing except me and God. There was silence. A silence so deep and powerful that I knew I was okay. I was wrapped in a warm duvet, cosseted and loved while just being. I'm the spiritual spark inside a body that has endured much pain and many treatments.

My body needs time to heal and repair itself. My mind goes in and out of fear and insecurity, but underneath it all I see the illusion. I'm grateful for another day, another moment, and all it brings.

It's almost weird that I wouldn't want anyone to have this experience and go through the treatments which have racked my body. However, this is something that was given to me and allowed me to see that I am healthy inside. My physical body might be unwell, my cells had multiplied, but I am always okay, no matter what. My mental health is intact and unbroken, untainted. My essence, core, spirit is always all right. I know from my experience at the beginning of this journey that there is something that is all encompassing, all embracing, and in charge of everything. This something is formless and form, and nothing but everything. It is whole and perfect and I'm a part of it; we all are. We are all pure love, uncontaminated by our personal thoughts, at its highest level. You too are included – don't sit in the corner and think it's good for me or him but not for you. We are all one, all part of the whole.

From my experience, I have felt great times of such deep connection with the oneness that it has almost taken my breath away. It is awesome that the silence had a depth of feeling I had not touched before. In those moments there was nothing to do or be. It just was. The silence made me understand that I need to lean into life and it will take me where I am meant to go.

In times of great pain during chemotherapy, I knew

deep down that the only thing that made me feel sorry for myself and wonder more about death than life was my thinking. The illusion got hold of me and trapped me sometimes. I knew it would stop and my perspective would change. It's a lifesaver, knowing that the occasions when it all appeared to be insurmountable and painful vanished into thin air from one moment to the next.

The knowing came from deep within me. I can't say it was from anywhere in particular in my body. Far deeper than body deep, touching my soul and my essence, my core, brushing lightly with its touch. I felt secure, held, loved and warmth. It was at the very heart of my being.

There is a lightness to life that shows itself with grace. It's subtle and tender. Loving and powerful. I love the fact that we can live with grace and gratitude. It gave me permission to be gentle with myself, not to demand I do better but to have the confidence to live from a place of the unknown. Everything I thought I knew was thrown out of the window.

The unknown was a scary place full of pit holes that I couldn't and wouldn't see. It looked like an ugly frightening monster. When we hold on tight, our knuckles become white from the pain of holding on. The harder we keep latched on, the more our knuckles hurt and we begin to lose grip. How much easier is it to accept that we have no idea what is going to happen? We cannot predict the future or change the past, but we can live more in the present moment and let go of our fears.

Love is the opposite of separateness for it embraces us and has no need for differences of interests or anything else that is personal. Love at its purest is formless. We cannot touch it. It isn't tangible. We are not taught to love. We are love. It is the fabric of our makeup, our deep inner self. Love is intuitive. If I take hot water and pour it into four different cups, it is just four cups of hot water. Add into one a black-berry flavor tea, into another mint, the third a strawberry tea bag and the last a lemon, then they are all different flavors. They started out the same, but once we dipped our personal preference into the hot water, it took a different flavor, color, taste.

That is what we all do with our life. We are given thoughts that are completely neutral, just like the hot water, and then we add our own flavors, our own personal opinions and beliefs into the mix. Our essence, our soul, is untouched by anything. Hope and potential are always on the horizon, constantly and unwaveringly available always to all of us.

I had an insight over twelve years ago, which was so profound I changed in an instant. I kept looking behind me, wondering when the old Sue Lachman would return, but she didn't. I came to a new awareness. I understood that without me needing to do anything, my thoughts change, and the reason for my misery and discomfort was because of what I was thinking at the time. That made me see that if my thoughts were different, I might no longer be in that place but would have moved on to something else.

The strangest thing, though, is that I am blindsided sometimes when something comes up for me, and I go down the rabbit hole, chasing the rabbit that isn't there. It appears as if I have lost that initial insight and I'm back to where I was before. Then I reconnect, the ground stops moving so fast, and I love and am kind and gentle to myself. It was me that chased the rabbit, me that dove down into the hole, and that's fine. It's human. We all do it without realizing. We all create our own reality via thought and take off like a hare.

I settle as I know that, without fail, my feelings are always only telling me what I am thinking in that moment. Relief washes over me when I see with that reminder that my awareness shoots up and I can see the same view from a different angle. I have been honored and grateful for the ability to bring people together and guide others to the same understanding of this profound, beautiful but simple acceptance of how life works.

One of the parts I enjoyed most was creating something from nothing, and out of nowhere people came from all over. Bringing speakers from America and England ensured that a greater amount of people could join together and be one in the feeling of love and hope. Suddenly everything changed and although my heart wanted to bring another speaker over, I knew it would not be possible.

I had started a conversation with Dr. Jack Pransky, who I met at the Viva Event in Albir, Spain, run by Sheela Masand and Sue Pankiewitz. I loved the idea and the ease of the event, which allows for people to come together to connect, have fun and learn about the Three Principles that explain the fabric and foundation of the innate health of each and every human being.

One year had already passed without organizing a seminar and I didn't want yet another year to pass. I encouraged my friend and colleague Raizel to take on the job of discussing and bringing Jack over to Israel as the key speaker. However, my jealousy surfaced. My body was incapable of doing all the difficult tasks that I had been able to co-ordinate on my own in the past, but my head and my heart did not want to let go. That meant that I felt acutely uncomfortable every time anyone mentioned that this was the first conference in Israel.

Technically it was indeed going to be the first conference, as before I had run seminars. The first few years the speakers spoke on their own, although more recently I had started working toward my dream of making it more like a conference; I wanted to ask local people to speak. This was my dream, not anyone else's, and I was loath to let it go, but let it go I had to. I could not physically do much to help.

Raizel excelled in all my hopes for a successful first conference, but something still bothered me. I wanted recognition and it seemed that everyone had forgotten that I started all this here. I was the brave one who paid out to bring people over and held my breath. I was the one who brought in enough people to fill a hall to capacity and have a waiting list. But then I saw that it wasn't anything to do with me, or Raizel for that matter.

June 3rd

I heard someone speak today at the first annual conference in Israel. She said she is the weather. She, we, all go in
and out of rain, wind, sun and whatever else the weather
brings. It changes in the blink of an eye and can stay for
minutes, hours or days. That is how our thinking goes. One
minute it's raining, the next it's just drizzle and with a light
breeze that's pleasant and welcome, gently touching my
face. Is this her personally speaking? Do you mean gently
touching our faces?

Believe me, being originally from England I know all
about the weather. It's often the first thing we talk about,
and as for rain, well, understanding that is an art, a skill.
Each type of rain has a different form. Sheet rain comes in
sheets, not stopping. A rainstorm comes out of the blue,
wets the land, and then as quickly as it comes, it goes.

June 10th – FB post

One year ago yesterday, 9th June 2017, my hand automatically went to do a breast self-examination. It wasn't something I did regularly but I had asked God the day before to show me what He wanted me to do now with my work, my life.

I got my answer loud and clear. Breast cancer. I slowed down more than I ever thought possible (I thought I had done that all before). I've spent the last year in pain (but not suffering). I've seen love and peace and although I am not done with treatment quite yet I can say I am done with the 'ugly' stuff.

Thanks to all of you for your prayers, your love and even though most of you are virtual, for your support and being there with me. I am slowly seeing a new normal.

GETTING BACK to normal as I knew it before is not happening. A new normal means that life has changed and I need to adjust to that. Go with the flow, so to speak, and accept that my body might not quite ever be the same as it was before treatment. Mentally I have certainly changed, grown.

Before I was introduced to the Three Principles my mind whirred all the time. I spent my life wondering what others thought of me and seeking approval. I felt self-conscious most of the time and believed that I needed to prove something to others and myself.

Life changed with my learning, understanding and deepening of seeing how life really works. The noises in my head became less intrusive, even though they were still there sometimes. They became less intense and I started to feel a weight off my mind. I thought I had slowed down. I had, but clearly this tap on my shoulder was to give me another lesson that I hadn't seen coming.

I stopped work the day we went to see the nurse in the oncology department. One minute I was busy, running around, speaking to people, organizing seminars and webinars. The next, a wall dropped in front of me. I had to stop. I had to slow down. There was nowhere to go, nothing to do, no one to be except me. To be myself.

As suddenly as I stopped, life started again once I began to heal from the radiotherapy. Thoughts started coming into my head at a furious rate and I felt caught up in life again. I needed a reminder, and I appealed to a group on Facebook for someone to point me in a different direction, guide me gently to see something else.

June 10th – FB post

I've been on a crazy adventure this year. Yesterday marked the one year mark of having breast cancer. I have through it all learned to slow down even more. I have also realized that I learn at my most vulnerable and when I am raw and honest about things.

I see that I need recognition all the time for past accomplishments. When I write or say it, it sounds ridiculous. I would love to see something different and not get so upset when someone says they're doing things and I immediately think, hang on I started all this, if it wasn't for me... Please don't tell me it's my ego. I know that intellectually. Eeeekkkk it's out there now.

I PUT myself out there as vulnerably as I dared and Deborah, a virtual Facebook friend, reached out to me. She asked if I would like to have a chat with her about my Facebook post and I took her up on her kind offer.

Her opening words were something about what's going on. And the floodgates opened. I sat there with tears rolling, speaking or rather slobbering my way through a conversation. I told her about my husband going, and touched on why I was fearful of the coming week without him. I hadn't even believed that this was an issue, that it was in the back of my mind.

I explained about feeling insulted that I was not recognized as being the initial and only person who had been organizing seminars and workshops for years before others were in Israel able to speak on the same Three Principles.

Deborah sat and listened until I finished, blew my nose and wiped my tears. She told me a story about her lawn mower. I don't know if this is exactly what she said, but this is my version, what I heard in the story.

Deborah has a big garden that requires mowing with a large machine. It was broken, so she had been using an old hand machine instead. The land was so large that she would have to deal with it in thirds, but by the time she finished the third part, she needed to start again as the grass she first mowed had already grown high. I had no idea why she was telling me about her lawn mower, but listened to her with interest and an open mind. Each time something popped into my head I realized that I was not listening, mainly because I was thinking of something of the past or the future. That in itself indicated that I was not listening to Deborah but to what was playing in the movie in my head.

She decided to take the lawn mower for a service on her way to visit her mother, something she felt she should have done during the winter months. The engineer told her it was scrap and she should throw it out. He mentioned that the skirt around the base of the machine was torn and impossible to repair. Likely it was dangerous too, but she didn't want to throw away a machine that worked to buy something that was costly and didn't have the same engine capacity.

When she mentioned it to her brother-in-law he said he could take a look at it. He was sure he could fix it and set about the work. He took the skirt off and replaced it with something he built and even painted to look like an original. The skirt had been held together with all the grass cuttings and without that would have fallen off.

Something clicked inside me. I am not sure how to put it into words and I have come to see that sometimes when something touches me deep inside, as dare I call it, at soul level, I am lost for words to describe what has happened.

I saw that the grass is all my thoughts holding something in place that is old and not useful anymore. Things work, life continues, but with all that stuff stuck around the skirt, all those thoughts, I wasn't allowing for something new to come in, to be formed and for me to be renewed. It was simple, yet gentle, a wiping away of the grass cuttings, hundreds and thousands of them stuck in the system which was holding me together but not in a helpful way. Maybe some would have thrown me on the scrap heap too, dismissed me as useless: that's the way life works, you are no good, you will never see through it, just live with it. But my deep listening and her story touched a chord without me needing to work out what the story meant or what significance it had. I am eternally grateful to you, Deborah.

Frank went to London and I felt very alone. It was the first time I had been left in the house during the day on my own since my diagnosis. Maybe I was scared that something might happen and I would have to deal with it without the support I was used to. I don't know.

JUNE **20**th

The speaker came on to stage in a wheelchair. I was shocked to see her now compared to our last encounter three years ago. A well-known and inspirational speaker, Tammy was respected and sought after in our community. She had given so many people a will to live.

This evening was the first time I went out to an event. I had avoided crowds for a year. One of the speakers moved me and helped me see something I had found difficult to put into words.

A carer, one of her daughters and two young ladies accompanied Tammy on to the stage. On her lap was a large sheet of what looked like Perspex with letters written on it, each in its own square. This is how Tammy communicates with her family, her carers, the world. A speech that she made which took about three minutes to read took her forty minutes to map using the sheet.

That in itself is remarkable. Tammy has amyotrophic lateral sclerosis (ALS), a motor neuron disease affecting the nerves which control muscle movement. It leads to muscle weakness and ultimately can be fatal. The last time I met Tammy she was able to converse with me and others around her, although her speech was slow. Now she is unable to speak except through the people who notice her eye movements, painstakingly watch her eyes and write down the letters, making words and eventually sentences.

Her speech for me was monumental in one particular sentence. This is what I heard her say: "You may think I am not here but I am. I am living very serenely." I know that feeling, I understand that space. And although I cannot claim to ever be in the same position that Tammy is in, I have had a glimpse of the serenity, the stillness and tranquility which she alludes to. I have had moments of being completely content with being at one with my essence and understanding there is nothing I need to do, nowhere I need to get to. Be. In the moment. I thank you, dear Tammy, for helping me to be more aware of the gift I was given in the middle of what could have been turmoil and suffering. We are all gifted with the ability to step into that space. To feel pure love and to be content with what is.

I was invited to give a talk to the ladies of a club I used to frequent. I was unable to attend while I had cancer, but many of the club members visited or phoned me. I was excited but had no idea what to say. After running some ideas around in my head, I decided that I would leave it and knew that whatever would come out of my mouth would be right.

Dropping the idea of needing to say something in particular, and letting go of the thinking I believed I needed to get my message across, were both really helpful. I was free to go and be myself instead of who I thought I needed to be. That's not to say I didn't start off with all that on my mind, but it quickly dropped away to leave room for me to have a quieter mind.

We crowded into a room that was unprepared for us. I looked around the room at everyone busying themselves, getting tea and coffee and some food. More chairs were needed. In the corner of the room, one of the ladies called for people to choose from a menu for an end of year brunch. This is life, back into it, full swing.

Starting to speak, I went in with very little on my mind for the outcome. I was weak today and my voice was quiet and had a slight tremor to it. I had no idea what I was going to say but the words started to flow out of me. I looked around the room and I saw people moved by my retelling of my experience. I too was moved to assure them that, no matter what, I was okay during the whole year. No matter what I had gone through physically it was just that...a physical experience which mostly did not get me down or wear me thin. I admitted that once, when I was in terrible pain, I wanted the Earth to open and swallow me. I didn't know if I wanted to live.

One of the women called out that I was lucky to have the support of my husband. She was right. But I knew it has nothing to do with luck. I knew that if I had expectations of how I thought something should be then I might well be disappointed. My attitude towards whatever was done for me was one of gratitude. Having a sour face or feeling hard done by would come from me and had nothing to do with my husband, or anyone else.

July 4ᵗʰ

Back for some more physiotherapy today. The physiotherapist is trained specifically in lymphedema. She
massaged my arm, the back of my neck and my breast. The
scar is still sore and the lump inside is hard. Thankfully,
though, I have full movement of my arm, although it swells
in the heat and when I use it too much.

My sister called and we spoke for a long time. She
started to tell me how brave I am and how she finds it
amazing that I had a sense of humor through it all. She
reminded me of when I went for treatment one day. It had
been raining and the roads were slippery. When it rains in
Israel it is freezing cold, too. I went in to the oncology
department, found a seat and went back to have my blood
taken and the cannula put in. When I returned, I noticed
that the seats, usually all taken at that time, were mostly
empty. I said to Frieda, my nurse, "Where is everyone? Are
they all dead?"

She laughed and told me that people often don't come

early when it rains. It takes them longer to get out and get themselves together for treatment.

Yes, I have a weird sense of humor, but it reminded me of when I took my dad to one of his appointments in the oncology ward in London. When he went in, he looked around and saw his friend not there. He turned to me and said, "It's okay – he's probably dead."

From what he said, I had this feeling that death is not bad. It's part of life, and so I could joke about it, knowing underneath that even though maybe one or two might never come back to their seats, it was unlikely that fifteen of them had left this Earth all at once.

My sister told me that I never once complained. Yes, I might have said I was tired or something hurt or I didn't want something, but I never complained. That was interesting, as I saw it differently. I believed that I hadn't stopped complaining about this or that and I wished I was able to withstand it all. We all see things differently, and we see our side of the story often with a blacker hue to it.

JULY 5th

Life is returning to whatever it was before. But not as it was before. I was busy ironing, though I have now discovered that putting it all in the tumble drier means there is less ironing. I used to iron everything except the underwear; my mum used to iron even that. When I iron, my mind goes from one thing to another, and today something came into my head that stopped me.

I knew it already, but when it pierces deeper, penetrates to my soul, it makes a deep-seated impression. I understood at a basic level that the Universe has our backs. Always. This insight came to me this morning after reading a post on one of the Facebook groups I'm on. The woman who posted has three children, a husband, a slew of animals, works a forty hour a week corporate job as well as finding time to do five hours a week freelance writing. She wants to write a certain amount of words a day to become a serious writer and author and build her empire. She has had two deaths in her family recently, but her focus is on only being able to write 1000 words a day, which is below her goal.

She writes that she can't get in the right place mentally. Wow. I noticed that the universe is calling out to her to slow down. It is gently tapping her on her shoulder. Reminding her as it does to all of us that we can be kind to ourselves. We can take a break. We do not need to beat ourselves up all the time. We are the ones who set the goals; that means we can change them accordingly. They're not written in stone and it doesn't mean we are a bad person or need to go for therapy.

Sometimes, as I discovered, we need to take a step back. Wait. Draw breath. Look around. Maybe something different will occur to us. Maybe it won't and that doesn't matter. That's fine too. But taking time out just puts things in perspective, helps us to observe from the sidelines and move on.

JULY 13th

I only noticed that it was Friday 13th when I looked at my calendar. Yosef is excited at the idea of buying a new car. He has researched and today he wants to go to the showroom to have a proper look at the models he's investigated. I told him I couldn't go but Frank would go with him. On reflection, I decided that my family, my children are important to me. I want to be interested in what interests them so I decided to go after all.

We left the house later than expected but managed to spend time going in and out of the cars, looking at the steering wheels and all the knobs and buttons. Checking out the screen on the dashboard, let alone the seats and leg room, all took time. At the end, Yosef questioned a sales person. We left armed with information and a beautiful shiny brochure.

Alister, Yael and their children had asked if they could come for the weekend. On the way back we picked them up, except for Yael, who would follow by bus as she was working. Nearly home, we stopped for petrol. Then we stopped for Yosef to buy some beer that was on special offer. That's when it happened. A tanker took the corner too sharply and took the side of our car off while we all sat in there. Thank God no one was hurt, but it gave me a jolt. Life is so precious: in one moment something can change and life could be snuffed out.

JULY 16th

I have been complaining that Frank can't hear too well so I decided to keep him company and sort out a hearing test for both of us. I wanted to prove that he can't hear me, but to my absolute shock, I'm the one with the hearing deficiency. According to the test, I need hearing aids in both ears. On returning home I discovered that chemotherapy and radiotherapy can cause hearing loss.

When will things settle?

July 16th – FB post

That sneaky chemo and radiotherapy.

Now I need two hearing aids...what did you say? Yup two, hearing loss in both ears.

We wanted a second opinion before we bought expensive hearing aids. First stop was to see the nurse and get the necessary paperwork for a further hearing test in a soundproof room. Not something that was done in the first test as both Frank and I could hear noises coming from a room above us.

As we walked towards the doctor's clinic, Frank said, "If you swallow the pills instead of stuffing them in your ears you might hear me."

I was cracking up about that. He actually told a joke. Or maybe he always did and I could never hear him. Hmmmm.

I ave a further hearing test in a couple of weeks and then I'm off to see an ear, nose and throat specialist for her recommendations.

JULY 17th

The physiotherapist, during one of our first meetings, measured some of my fingers, wrist and arm at strategic points and made a note. She followed up a week later with more measurements and then announced that I would need to wear a sleeve and glove to keep the swelling down.

In extreme weather the heat or cold can affect my arm. I intend to fly out of the country in the near future for a speaking engagement, and the flight can cause swelling and pain in the arm and fingers. Or so the physiotherapist told me. It was a no brainer to decide to have a sleeve and half glove if nothing else, and to keep my arm safe during a flight. It was going to take approximately two weeks for them to be manufactured for me. Each sleeve and glove is made according to precise measurements. It was cheaper than expected as I ordered a glove without the fingers. That's good, now I have enough for a deposit for my hearing aids.

Scanning through Facebook posts, I noticed an organization in America provides holidays for people with cancer at minimal cost. My mind drifted to the thought of getting away and not needing to prepare anything. Just to take off and be free for a little while from all the appointments for me and Chaya Gittel.

I doubted that anything was set up in Israel. How wrong I was.

On a recent visit to the hospital, Chops (everyone asks her how she got the name and her reply is always the same: "Don't ask!" and she laughs), the oncologist's secretary, handed Frank a leaflet. Their website says: 'Give cancer time out. Go on a healing holiday today'. I am in awe of the set up. We registered today but have no idea where we will end up going. Such fun, an adventure.

On checking out the website, I cried at the kindness of all the people giving up their holiday homes, a room in a bed and breakfast or even hotel rooms. Some have donated times in their bed and breakfasts. Many of these accommodations are in tranquil, relaxing places.

FIFTEEN

AUGUST 2018

August 7th – FB post

It was a no go as the needle didn't go in and all the time she huffed and puffed and then I could see the tears. She cried out in pain as the needle was removed and repositioned farther down towards her wrist. Once again, her face wrinkled and the pain was evident in her face.

I thank God mine was a little easier but it's never wonderful.

I couldn't take my eyes off the unfolding scene. I felt detached yet in the moment, understanding where the woman's pain was coming from. There is no doubt in my mind that the pain to her was real. But she had already predicted what might happen before the needle had even gone into her veins.

Often, we base our experience of what will happen on what has happened. It's natural that this occurs. But what if we could look at it differently, be willing to see that maybe it might not be the same as before? Perhaps.

Now I wait for the medication to be ordered. At least

nowadays it only takes about two to three hours instead of all day.

Tomorrow is another procedure for my daughter. We have to be in the hospital by 7:30 a.m. Then finally I get to see the ENT to decide about my hearing.

I HAVE a friend who told me a lovely story about her experience of something that happened had changed. My friend lived abroad while her mother lives in London. My friend's husband had gone to London to work for the week when she got news that her maternal grandmother had died.

She wanted to go to London to be with her mother but had two very boisterous boys with her. Her past experience had always shown her that to fly anywhere with her children was challenging, to say the least. She was loath to fly alone to do something that with her husband had always felt such a chore and difficult. She called her husband, asking him to fly home so he could join her in going back to London. Needless to say, her husband refused and told her she could do it alone.

In that moment, she knew that she was basing something that might never happen on something that had happened in the past. That meant she had put it all in a neat little box and closed it all up. There was no room for maneuvering. It had to happen, in her mind, the way it had always happened before.

Seeing that, she decided to let things happen naturally without managing anything. She booked the flights, packed the cases with little effort and headed towards the airport with her two boys. At the airport she saw an old friend, who was on the same flight and gave her a helping hand with the boys on the flight.

Her experience was completely different to the one she thought she would have. She had made up how it would be without allowing it to be different.

I couldn't help but wonder. If the woman hadn't been looking so closely into her past, perhaps her experience this time might not be as it had before. Perhaps it might be similar but not the same. It's an idea to sit with.

August 9th – FB post

It's tiring sitting in a hospital from just after 7 a.m until we left early afternoon. Chaya Gittel had her procedure. No results until the next one on 21st August.

I thought it was hilarious that the minute she was more awake in the recovery room, she started looking around and asking about this one and that one. Nosey like her mum. She was my excuse to look too, lol.

So much gratitude to Avital Chevern who once again came with us and helped with everything which made it so much easier for us. How can we ever thank you?!

There was a young woman there with her father, or might have been her husband, and son. The boy was very active. They were running after him. He kept trying to take out the cannula they put in which was difficult enough to get there in the first place. No differences between us. Both families with a child with special needs. We smiled and nodded to each other, understanding the other. One Jew, one Arab.

Saw the ENT – she told me definitely the chemo helped the hearing loss. My decision to see if hearing aids will help.

I LOVE my daughter's natural curiosity. She is genuinely interested in what is going on around her. One time when she first started having seizures, she was taken from the accident and emergency in the hospital. She loved being in there, where there was life and interesting people moving around her. You could see how she felt part of life, connected to everyone around her.

How cool. I can actually hear conversations better now. I was straining to hear in some environments. Often, I had to ask people to repeat themselves. After three hearing tests and speaking to the specialist, we ordered two hearing aids.

August 28th – FB post

Sitting waiting for treatment at the hospital. Have been here now for seventy-five minutes. Still waiting to be hooked up to the clear stuff in the plastic bag.

I love being able to hear everything. The best fun is being able to press my left aid to answer the phone, heh heh. People look at me wondering who I'm speaking to.

My daughter had her last (we hope) procedure, so waiting for the results. We hope she won't need an operation and they will just keep her on medication.

Best news – the nurse just told me next one is my last intravenous treatment. She's gone off to count and make sure. I am so emotional about this I'm crying with joy.

Will only have one pill to take every day for best part of another four and a half years. No, not that pill lol.

THERE'S an incredible feeling of relief. I'm nearly finished with the regular hospital visits. I have a sense of deep peace and happiness. I'm full of joy.

SIXTEEN

SEPTEMBER TO DECEMBER 2018

September 17th – FB post

Mixed emotions today. I'm excited that this might be the last infusion I need. On the other hand, I feel nervous butterflies. For over a year since finding the lump in my breast in June 2017 I have been looked after, loved, felt the full support of nurses, a surgeon, an oncologist, my friends and my amazing family and now it will all fall away. But there's something magical that I glimpsed.

It's also soooo exciting...

IT'S VERY STRANGE. Suddenly I feel alone. Nowhere to go every so often. No one to see. I can do what I want without the restraint of needing to be at an appointment. On one hand, it's a sense of freedom, but on the other it's a little scary. I'm alone to continue the journey deeper into the unknown without the reassurance from professionals. They're there but no longer there.

Every little thing I do, it's as if it's the first time. I

remember a similar feeling after I lost my dad and then my mum. We sat in mourning for a week, and when we first got up after the time was finished, life seemed to be in slow motion. It was as if life was starting again and it took time to get to get going. After being cosseted for such a long period of time, although I was surrounded by my family and friends, I thought I was alone. An emptiness encompassed me and I felt fearful and unsure of what I should do. Then I remembered that the feeling of being alone was just something I was experiencing at the moment. It passed as each day went on.

That feeling of loss is all made up. I hadn't lost anything. My security or insecurity is all down to me. I once heard Linda Pransky, another Three Principles facilitator, say that we are either having secure or insecure thoughts. It is so basic and so simple, but we complicate it.

October 3rd – FB post

My first time out of country for a year and a half. So looking forward to being at this special event.

Come and join us. It is such fun.

I was invited to speak in a breakout session at the annual Viva Event in Spain. We planned the trip, making sure all the connecting flights would not have too long a stopover but enough time to reach the next flight.

But as we know, the best laid plans and all that. The airline changed the flight carrier, which meant we only had an hour between the first and second flight. Wouldn't you know it? The first flight was delayed, and consequently, even though I tried running to the gate, they had closed it and taken our luggage off. Eventually they magically found two places on the flight that we had booked anyway, but without our luggage. For some unknown reason we were not registered as having taken that flight, which had consequences on the way back.

OCTOBER 24th

Sometimes I feel as if I am on a see-saw. One day I am up in the air and then next it is my daughter, Chaya Gittel. In between everything we still had the diagnosis of Moyamoya hanging over our heads, and what that would mean. I wanted to get to the bottom of her behavioral issues, which I was sure were due to a mixture of this diagnosis and her thyroid issues rather than her just misbehaving.

My brave little heroine had two procedures, which meant she had to be sedated on both occasions. We knew she would be unable to be still during the procedure and opted for a general anesthetic. She came round each time with that fighting spirit and that thirst to want to see and know what was going on around her.

November 6th –FB post

Just on way home from a magical time at Viva. Yesterday we made sure our flights were secure and that we would have kosher food for the long part of the journey. We were told as we didn't take our flight last Thursday from Madrid to Alicante there was no return flight – they cancelled it. After telling them we had definitely been on the flight to Alicante they finally agreed to reinstate us on the return flight.

Now to tackle the kosher food part. Hmmm, she said we had to call next day. Well that would be too late. So, I used FB messenger. They told me they have one kosher meal booked for my husband. I explained we needed two meals and we had ordered them ages ago. Finally, we got two meals.

Then what happens? First flight this morning was over an hour late so we missed the connecting flight. Now I'm hoping those kosher meals don't get upset we can't eat them lol.

IT SEEMS that we were meant to have a challenging journey both ways. We both knew that although we would not get back home until the following day, we were okay. As we had missed the onward flight from Madrid to Tel Aviv, we waited in the airport for approximately nine hours. Throughout it all neither of us got flustered or angry. We knew that the only thing that could annoy us were the thoughts we were having about what was unfolding. Those thoughts just came and went as we weren't entertaining them. We didn't take any of them seriously so they left.

Since that excursion I have been declared to be in full remission. It looks like the treatment left me with a heart problem, which is being tested extensively. I am hopeful that soon we will get to the bottom of it. Although my breathing is labored when even walking a few steps, it has not stopped my determination to live life to its fullest.

December 6th – FB post

First mammogram today since treatment and operations then off to see oncologist. What stories can I make up today before I even see anyone hmmmm?

WE MADE our way to the hospital. I was unsure what to

expect from the mammogram, which was the first appointment of the day. In the past, mammograms and being squashed under a machine, even for a couple of seconds, were not fun. I started to wonder what the pain would be like now I only had a third of my original right breast.

I had spent some time in the days preceding the appointment examining my right breast to see what might be in there. I think I was trying to preempt the situation, and I managed to convince myself at one stage that there was a lump and a tumor had started to grow again. Luckily, I read that after surgery there were more unusual bumps and lumps, so the voice in my head quieted. But then there was the pain under my arm, and I was sure I could feel small nodules. Maybe they were new tumors growing? I knew that I was making up a whole story. I was imagining things.

I stopped wasting my time with my fairytales and took each moment as it came. I had dealt with stuff before and if I needed to I would again. Worrying about something that I couldn't control and might come to pass would be fruitless. A waste of my precious time. I would much rather be doing things I enjoy. The mammogram was not nearly as painful as I first thought but I had to have an ultrasound before I got the results. I could see the doctor smiling, and then the best words came out of his mouth: "It's all clear." I was elated.

Professor Cherney, always smiling, always happy to see everyone, greeted me and the first thing he said was that the mammogram was clear. He reassured me that my doctor was right in sending me to him. I had begun to think I was a fraud, in particular as the pain in my left arm had improved. He examined my shoulder and the two main spots of my pain and determined I would need a blood test and a PET CT scan. I felt reassured by the appointment and realized how important it was to report any new ache or pain. I was more sure that the pain I felt was not cancer, but the oncologist said we should get to the bottom of whatever it might be.

December 10th – FB post

AMAZING NEWS!

Mammogram is clear. Just had blood test and need a PET CT scan for my back/shoulder just to see what it is.

Once again will be pumped with nuclear stuff and then put into a special room while we all go off the Geiger counter grid.

THE PET CT scan went well. I knew the procedure, so it seemed a little easier. I just wish the young guy putting the cannula in knew about the bruises he left me with. In went the needle, but not without some searing pain in my arm. I then watched him move the needle around inside my arm.

"Do you not bleed so well?"

What? I didn't even understand what he meant until I saw that not a drop of blood was coming from the area where he put the needle. I thought that very strange, as the phlebotomist locally had easily taken blood from me on the other day. After what seemed like ages, he took the needle out, telling me it was in my vein but there was no blood there. It is still black and blue a week later.

He proceeded to attack my hand to find a place to go in. I'm here though to tell the story. The Geiger counter played its part and now it's time for the result.

. . .

DECEMBER **24**th

My results are in and very encouraging, in the words of the oncologist. He is pretty sure that although there is something lurking in the picture, it is not malignant. He wants me to have an MRI, but it is just a matter of course so he can get to the bottom of the pain.

I swayed between believing everything was okay and that I had more tumors. One of the things I decided, though, was that I didn't want to waste my time worrying. We have that opportunity every minute of the day. We often get caught up and don't see that we can choose to be here rather than there.

SEVENTEEN
CONNECTION

Many years and five children later, the memory of the benign cyst was buried deep inside and nearly forgotten.

Most people don't know what to say when they hear you have cancer. It's not easy. Some have told me that their mother or great aunt had cancer and they are thriving now. They survived.

There are others who have flooded me with information about this new treatment or that new drug, let alone what to eat and even what to wash with. All the advice and good intentions are overwhelming, along with the knowledge that people care and want to help. If they only realized the amount of different ideas that come your way, I'm sure many would refrain from adding to the pile.

Then you feel like everyone wants to cross the road and avoid you. It must be difficult to know what to say to people because the C word has connotations, but please act normally. Just be compassionate, wonder how you might like to be spoken to if in this situation. Don't worry, it's not catching, it won't jump from me to you.

It's strange but at first people didn't visit me or speak to me – it was as if I knew no one. My closest friends were there, knowing how to connect, although still, to a certain extent, they kept their distance, maybe wondering if I was up to it and how I was reacting to all the news.

I know you all wanted to do the best for me, but sometimes I needed to tell a stranger or someone not so close to me how awful I physically felt and the pain of the treatments. I wanted to be listened to at times and for you to be there for me. Someone called me, someone who had come quite regularly to our house for the weekend, a friend of our boys. He apologized for not calling sooner but said, "I'm sorry I didn't call sooner, I just have no idea what to say to you."

Now I understand this. I have children with special needs and I have seen people actually cross the road to avoid me. The admittance of not knowing what to say, though, was refreshing to hear. I honestly wouldn't have known what to say to someone before my diagnosis, either. I wouldn't have known what to say to people before having my own children with Down syndrome. I would say, though, that rather than people feeling the need to walk on another side of the road because they feel awkward and don't know what to say...just tell someone you don't know what to say! I felt remembered. There is no right or wrong list of things to say, because we all do things that make sense to us at the time.

I know there have been times in my life when I wanted and had the intention to visit someone who wasn't well or maybe had lost a parent but the time passed, it didn't happen. Just know though that it's never too late, there's no need to be embarrassed that you didn't call or visit earlier. I remember one time when living in London, a friend's daughter was unwell and I had in mind to make her a meal.

The thought occurred to me more than once and I even made the shepherd's pie in my head, but in reality, it never got made.

Life seems to take over and good intentions go out the window. I finally got the food to her when one of my sons had a Bar Mitzvah and I asked the caterer, who happened to be her father, to make an individual pie. We all laughed, but it's easy to condemn people for not doing things we expect or hope they will do, even something as simple as making a meal for a family in need. On the other hand, I am very aware of my forgetfulness even when I have the best of intentions.

Maybe it all stems from this fear we have of the unknown, death. Cancer is for most of us the next step before the inevitable — death. It's no longer like that for so many. And no, I won't necessarily lose weight; those that do are possibly very sick. Sounds crazy, but a friend of mine told me that at least now I would lose some weight!

The drugs they put into my body brought me from being a healthy person to someone who was sometimes as weak as a kitten. The pain at times was relentless and excruciating, and physically I was drained. My body felt abused and broken. I was well before I started treatment.

Between all the pain, the unpleasant infusions, and enduring the hospital system, there were more than a fair share of fresh thoughts that buoyed me. Connection is something most of us seek. A conversation, sitting, listening, or being listened to, connects us all in different ways. We can have that feeling with ourselves too.

When I lived in London, I attended a meeting organized by a lady who wanted to help mothers of special needs children. I was invited to the meeting for two reasons: I have two children with Down syndrome and I helped parents of children with special needs to receive their rights from the municipality. The room was crammed with mothers eager to hear the plans for our children. We were excited, hopeful. We were hopeful the meeting would focus on offering us a chance of a break from the children maybe once or twice a week. For them to be taken out of the house for an activity. However, we were told a volunteer would be sent to our house to visit our children and play with them.

We explained that we needed someone to take our children out of the house for an hour, so we could be with our other children or spend time making supper without having to be on call all the time. That would relieve us and be more beneficial. But the lady, who was a mother herself although not of children with special needs, and her cohort of friends would not hear of it. They believed they knew what was best for us without wanting to listen. They stood firm in their belief and it all fell through. They rejected our proposal to take the children out of the house.

Listening to one another is so important. Even when we think we are listening, we often go into conversations with a preconceived idea or an agenda. Other times, mid-conversation we think we have the solution and have this burning need to state it. But that is not listening to the other person beyond their words, it is listening to ourselves.

Listening to others is one of the most profound experiences I have encountered. My husband used to travel a lot for business. Thankfully the journey from Israel to London is far less than to America, so not so difficult for him. Regular flying also helped to allay his fears. He would leave on a Sunday and return either

Thursday or Friday. He was tired, not just from the flight, but the week of non-stop work, often until late at night.

This particular week he stood no more than four feet from me. He took off his watch, placed it on our dining room table and began to have a conversation with me. This was a Friday morning and preparations still had to be completed for the Sabbath. But I listened to him. I know he talked about all the hard work he had to do and how he was occupied with clients.

While he talked, several things came into my head, starting with, "I hope he hurries, I still need to bake challahs". I realized I was not listening to Frank but to what was in my head, my thoughts. I returned to listening to him.

Other things came in my mind, like, "I wonder when he will stop talking because I need to sit, my legs are getting tired". If I stopped to get a chair I might break his train of thought, and in turn our connection. Each time something popped into my head, I naturally went back to listening. When I listened to him, I felt a deep connection with him. When I was thinking about something I needed to do in the future, or about me and my situation, there was no electric feeling. At the end, he stopped. There was silence. Then something occurred to me.

"I'm so sorry, I know that every Friday you bring me flowers but I never say thank you. I'm not always grateful."

"How did you know I thought that?" he replied.

It bubbled up from inside me. I'm going to call it wisdom that showed itself to me. We connected when I listened deeply to him, and I heard something that is not possible to describe as it is intangible.

With cancer came gifts. The gift of life, hearing the birds sing, seeing the blue sky and the trees swaying in the gentle breeze. I am alive! Seeing a smile from the volunteers who came to the oncology ward or the kind breast surgeon's nurse who often came to visit. The love shown throughout.

Listening deeply to everyone around me. The present of the present moment. The sheer joy and excitement of seeing my grandchildren. These are all the benefits to being alive and thanking God each day for another one. The best thing is that it's all free!

Knowing that there is nothing to fix is a comfort. Any bad feelings I have, I don't need to adjust or change them. I listened to my body rather than my head. I instinctively knew when to rest or when to eat. I saw the clouds outside move across the sky. Sometimes there were none to be seen. Just like the clouds, a bad feeling might move along and I didn't need to physically move it out of the way.

The brain is amazing. Chaya Gittel's brain found a new route for some of the blood vessels to travel through to ensure she had enough blood going to her head. The other part hadn't quite worked it out yet, but as a result they did not want to knock out any of the natural alignment the brain and vessels had worked out. The professional team decided not to operate at the moment. We were relieved.

I know you have navigated many changes in your life. Maybe while you were in the middle of it, it felt very dark and heavy, or maybe some of the changes were light and easy. But daily we all go through ordinary changes. Sometimes we navigate them gracefully and at other times we fall down and graze our knees or break a bone.

If there is any trick to understanding changes, it would be to see that they are inevitable. They come and go like the wind and the rain. They are random. When we see them for what they are, just a movement, a different maneuver to what we are expecting, then we are able to transition with ease. It is often our expectation of a situation that pulls us back. Expectations are assumptions we make about something in the future that might or might not happen. They take us away from the present moment.

We do not know what will happen from one moment to the next. As someone said to me not long after my cancer diagnosis, "You could just as easily get run over by a bus". Now that might be true or it might not. At first, I was incensed by this statement until I saw it differently. It's true: just because I have cancer it does not mean I'll die from it.

I know that when I step aside, then it all works out. It might not be the way I thought it should or would be, but still, it works out. Often I will look back and wonder how clever it was that this or that happened, knowing that in my wildest dream, I wouldn't have come to the same conclusion or certainly not in the same way. After all, I know only the small part of the puzzle, the part I can see.

EIGHTEEN

JANUARY 2019

January 30th – FB post

Do you know how many people have asked us if we are going alone...just me and him...to Orlando to see Mickey Mouse?

Yes it's just the two of us and I'm beyond excited.

When I was first diagnosed with breast cancer one of the things we talked about was to just do stuff. No waiting and putting it off until whenever.

So this is one of our dreams...to go back to Disney and have fun. Just the two of us spending time together.

AND THAT'S what we did. We spent over two weeks laughing and giggling. We spent time together in the magical kingdom, and went full circle from where my story started.

VIP CLUB

Rethinking Relationships

To say thank you for reading my book, I'd like to invite you to my exclusive VIP Club and give you *'Rethinking Relationships'* FREE

**To join go to
https://www.suelachman.com/rethinking-relationships/
And sign up.**

The best thing is it's completely FREE. You will never be spammed and can unsubscribe at any time

DID YOU ENJOY THIS BOOK?

YOU CAN HELP MAKE A DIFFERENCE

Reviews are the most powerful means when it comes to getting attention for my books.

Honest reviews of my books help bring them to the attention of readers who might be encouraged to explore the possibility of creating a shift in their perspective, learning more about the Three Principles and living life in a more relaxed, happy calm manner.

If you enjoyed this book, I would be grateful if you could spend a few minutes and write an honest review (as long or as short as you wish) on the book's Amazon page.

Thank you

ABOUT THE AUTHOR

Sue writes relatable, honest authentic books with a dash of humour. Supporting women navigate the ups and downs of life and feel inspired to live life fully.

She is wife to one and mom of five. She is often found pottering around the house doing things that she hadn't noticed was written in the fine print!

Born in London she has a Certificate of Education and a B.A. neither of which taught her about how life really works.

She was busy but all caught up in life and helping people. But she forgot to help herself first. She noticed friends who were depressed, alcoholics, or suffering from trauma, change before her eyes. They started to see that their past didn't need to get in the way of their happiness.

To find out more:

http://www.suelachman.com/about/

https://instagram.com/suelachman

https://www.facebook.com/SueLachmanAuthor

For my Family who I love with all my heart

ALSO BY SUE LACHMAN

Downs and Ups

Life Is A Kaleidoscope

Life Is A Kaleidoscope (Workbook)

Rethinking Relationships

Uncovering The Light Within

Printed in Great Britain
by Amazon